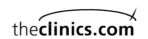

VETERINARY CLINICS

OF NORTH AMERICA

Small Animal Practice

Practical Applications and New
Perspectives in Veterinary Behavior

GUEST EDITORS
Gary M. Landsberg, DVM
Debra F. Horwitz, DVM

September 2008 • Volume 38 • Number 5

SAUNDERS

An Imprint of Elsevier, Inc.
PHILADELPHIA   LONDON   TORONTO   MONTREAL   SYDNEY   TOKYO

W.B. SAUNDERS COMPANY
A Division of Elsevier Inc.

1600 John F. Kennedy Boulevard · Suite 1800 · Philadelphia, PA 19103-2899

http://www.vetsmall.theclinics.com

VETERINARY CLINICS OF NORTH AMERICA:	Volume 38, Number 5
SMALL ANIMAL PRACTICE	ISSN 0195-5616
September 2008	ISBN-13: 978-1-4160-6374-2
Editor: John Vassallo; j.vassallo@elsevier.com	ISBN-10: 1-4160-6374-9

Veterinary Clinics of North America: Small Animal Practice (ISSN 0195-5616) is published bimonthly (For Post Office use only: volume 38 issue 5 of 6) by Elsevier Inc., 360 Park Avenue South, New York, NY 10010-1710. Months of issue are January, March, May, July, September, and November. Business and Editorial offices: 1600 John F. Kennedy Blvd., Suite 1800, Philadelphia, PA 19103-2899. Customer Service Office: 6277 Sea Harbor Drive, Orlando, FL 32887-4800. Periodicals postage paid at New York, NY and additional mailing offices. Subscription prices are $206.00 per year for US individuals, $327.00 per year for US institutions, $103.00 per year for US students and residents, $273.00 per year for Canadian individuals, $410.00 per year for Canadian institutions, $285.00 per year for international individuals, $410.00 per year for international institutions and $140.00 per year for Canadian and foreign students/residents. To receive student/resident rate, orders must be accompanied by name of affiliated institution, date of term, and the *signature* of program/residency coordinator on institution letterhead. Orders will be billed at individual rate until proof of status is received. Foreign air speed delivery is included in all *Clinics* subscription prices. All prices are subject to change without notice. **POSTMASTER**: Send address changes to *Veterinary Clinics of North America: Small Animal Practice*, Elsevier Periodicals Customer Service, 6277 Sea Harbor Drive, Orlando, FL 32887-4800. Customer Service: 1-800-654-2452 (US). From outside the United States, call 1-407-563-6020. Fax: 1-407-363-9661. E-mail: JournalsCustomerService-usa@elsevier.com.

Reprints. For copies of 100 or more of articles in this publication, please contact the Commercial Reprints Department, Elsevier Inc., 360 Park Avenue South, New York, NY 10010-1710. Tel.: 212-633-3812; Fax: 212-462-1935; E-mail: reprints@elsevier.com.

Veterinary Clinics of North America: Small Animal Practice is also published in Japanese by Inter Zoo Publishing Co., Ltd., Aoyama Crystal-Bldg 5F, 3-5-12 Kitaaoyama, Minato-ku, Tokyo 107-0061, Japan.

Veterinary Clinics of North America: Small Animal Practice is covered in *Current Contents/Agriculture, Biology and Environmental Sciences, Science Citation Index, ASCA, MEDLINE/PubMed (Index Medicus), Excerpta Medica,* and *BIOSIS.*

Printed in the United States of America.

ELSEVIER
SAUNDERS

VETERINARY CLINICS
SMALL ANIMAL PRACTICE

Practical Applications and New Perspectives in Veterinary Behavior

GUEST EDITORS

GARY M. LANDSBERG, DVM, Diplomate, American College of Veterinary Behaviorists; Diplomate, European College of Veterinary Behavioral Medicine (Companion Animals); Owner, North Toronto Animal Clinic; Doncaster Animal Clinic, Thornhill, Ontario, Canada

DEBRA F. HORWITZ, DVM, Diplomate, American College of Veterinary Behaviorists; Veterinary Behavior Consultations, St. Louis, Missouri

CONTRIBUTORS

LAURIE BERGMAN, VMD, Diplomate, American College of Veterinary Behaviorists; Metropolitan Veterinary Associates, Norristown, Pennsylvania

TERRY MARIE CURTIS, DVM, Diplomate, American College of Veterinary Behaviorists; College of Veterinary Medicine, University of Florida, Gainesville, Florida

JEAN DONALDSON, BSc, CPDT, Director, The San Francisco Society for the Prevention of Cruelty to Animals, The Academy for Dog Trainers, San Francisco, California

MARGARET M. DUXBURY, DVM, Diplomate, American College of Veterinary Behaviorists; Assistant Clinical Specialist, Behavior Service, University of Minnesota, Veterinary Medical Center, College of Veterinary Medicine, St. Paul, Minnesota

LORI GASKINS, DVM, Diplomate, American College of Veterinary Behaviorists; Assistant Professor, St. Matthew's University School of Veterinary Medicine, Cayman Islands, British West Indies

LORE I. HAUG, DVM, Diplomate, American College of Veterinary Behaviorists; South Texas Veterinary Behavior Services, Sugar Land, Texas

DEBRA F. HORWITZ, DVM, Diplomate, American College of Veterinary Behaviorists; Veterinary Behavior Consultations, St. Louis, Missouri

GARY M. LANDSBERG, DVM, Diplomate, American College of Veterinary Behaviorists; Diplomate, European College of Veterinary Behavioral Medicine (Companion Animals); Owner, North Toronto Animal Clinic; Doncaster Animal Clinic, Thornhill, Ontario, Canada

EMILY D. LEVINE, DVM, MRCVS, Diplomate, American College of Veterinary Behaviorists; Animal Emergency and Referral Associates, Fairfield, New Jersey

ANDREW U. LUESCHER, DVM, PhD, Diplomate, American College of Veterinary Behaviorists; European College of Veterinary Behavioral Medicine (Companion Animals); Associate Professor of Animal Behavior, and Director, Animal Behavior Clinic, Department of Veterinary Medicine, Purdue University School of Veterinary Medicine, Veterinary Clinical Sciences, West Lafayette, Indiana

AMY MARDER, VMD, CAAB, Director, Center for Shelter Dogs, Animal Rescue League of Boston, Boston, Massachusetts

DANIEL S. MILLS, BVSc, PhD, CBiol, MIBiol, CCAB, MRCVS, Diplomate, European College of Veterinary Behavioural Medicine (Companion Animals); Professor and RCVS Recognised Specialist in Veterinary Behavioural Medicine, and Head, Department of Biological Sciences, University of Lincoln, Lincoln, United Kingdom

KELLY MOFFAT, DVM, Diplomate, American College of Veterinary Behaviorists; VCA Mesa Animal Hospital, Mesa, Arizona

ILANA R. REISNER, DVM, PhD, Diplomate, American College of Veterinary Behaviorists; Department of Clinical Studies–Philadelphia, School of Veterinary Medicine, University of Pennsylvania, Philadelphia, Pennsylvania

LYNNE M. SEIBERT, DVM, PhD, Diplomate, American College of Veterinary Behaviorists; Owner, Veterinary Behavior Consultants, Kirkland, Washington

KERSTI SEKSEL, BVSc (Hons), MRCVS, FACVSc (Animal Behaviour), MA (Hons); Diplomate, American College of Veterinary Behaviorists; Diplomate, European College of Veterinary Behavioural Medicine (Companion Animals); Director, Sydney Animal Behaviour Service, Seaforth, New South Wales, Australia

JULIE SHAW, AS, RVT, Animal Behavior Technologist, Animal Behavior Clinic, Purdue University, West Lafayette, Indiana

BARBARA L. SHERMAN, PhD, DVM, Diplomate, American College of Veterinary Behaviorists; Clinical Associate Professor, Department of Clinical Sciences; and Director, Animal Behavior Service, Veterinary Teaching Hospital, North Carolina State University College of Veterinary Medicine, Raleigh, North Carolina

VETERINARY CLINICS
SMALL ANIMAL PRACTICE

Practical Applications and New Perspectives in Veterinary Behavior

Diagnosis and Management of Patients Presenting with Behavior Problems — 937

Lynne M. Seibert and Gary M. Landsberg

Behavior problems are among the most common concerns for veterinary clients, and veterinarians need to be comfortable diagnosing and treating these conditions. Knowledge of animal behavior by veterinarians is critical for effective treatment of behavior problems, recognition and diagnosis of medical conditions for which behavior signs prevail, proper handling of veterinary patients, prevention of abandonment and euthanasia, preservation of the companion animal–human bond, and prevention of mental suffering. Successful patient management requires taking a thorough behavioral history, understanding the mechanisms underlying behavior changes, developing appropriate treatment interventions, and, in some cases, pharmacologic therapy.

Handling Behavior Problems in the Practice Setting — 951

Gary M. Landsberg, Julie Shaw, and Jean Donaldson

The veterinary clinic plays a critical role in the prevention and treatment of behavior problems. If behavior problems do begin to emerge, the veterinary clinic can help determine who can advise and guide the owners most practically to improve or resolve the problem. This help might involve the veterinarian, a behavioral technician, a trained staff member, an appropriate trainer, or some combination of these persons. This article reviews how these professional roles might be integrated, depending on the complexity of the problem.

Preventing Behavior Problems in Puppies and Kittens — 971

Kersti Seksel

There are many common issues that owners find problematic with their puppy's or kitten's behavior, such as eliminating in inappropriate locations, chewing, mouthing, growling, and biting. Many of these issues can be prevented or managed by helping owners understand normal canine and feline behavior and by teaching the puppy and kitten socially acceptable behaviors. The focus always should be on rewarding acceptable behaviors rather than punishing unacceptable ones. Puppy

Preschool and Kitten Kindergarten classes are an ideal avenue to introduce pet owners to modern, humane ways to train and socialize their pets to be a valuable part of today's society.

Handling aggressive dogs and cats in the veterinary clinic can be frustrating, time consuming, and injurious for both employee and animal. This article discusses the etiology of the aggressive dog and cat patient and how best to approach these cases. A variety of handling techniques, safety products, and drug therapy are reviewed.

Management solutions offer a useful tool for owners faced with behavior issues in their pets. In some cases management will improve the behavior and allow control. In other situations it may be only the first step in treatment. By offering management solutions, veterinarians can help owners with problem pets and begin the road to recovery.

Aggression toward unfamiliar dogs and people is a common problem arising most commonly from fear and territoriality. A number of factors contribute to its development, including socialization deficits, hormones, and genetic and neurophysiologic components. These factors are discussed in this article, as are management and behavior modification approaches for controlling aggression.

Once clients make a decision to expand their family with children or pets, veterinarians can be instrumental in providing education and support to make the additions successful. Veterinarians should remind clients to make changes in the household well in advance of the new addition's arrival, to be patient, to make all introductions safe and controlled, and to reward good behavior. If problems arise, owners should be advised to separate those involved and get behavioral treatment as soon as possible. Through these simple steps, veterinarians can increase the likelihood that clients will be able to integrate new family members successfully.

VETERINARY CLINICS
SMALL ANIMAL PRACTICE

Vet Clin Small Anim 38 (2008) xi–xiii

VETERINARY CLINICS
SMALL ANIMAL PRACTICE

Preface

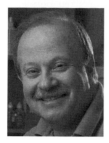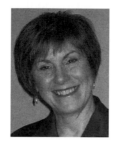

Gary M. Landsberg, DVM
Debra F. Horwitz, DVM

Guest Editors

I t has been over 25 years since the first *Veterinary Clinics of North America: Small Animal Practice* issue devoted to behavior, edited by Drs. Victoria Voith and Peter Borchelt, was published. In that time, the field of veterinary behavior has grown considerably. The field of veterinary behavior is now a recognized specialty with, at the time of writing, 46 board-certified diplomates of the American College of Veterinary Behaviorists, and it continues to grow. That first issue introduced the veterinary practitioner to some new concepts, and in some cases a new area of veterinary practice, and began a journey that has included several additional behavior issues in this series, with the latest coming to you today.

In this issue, we continue the tradition of helping practitioners focus on the importance of prevention, diagnosis, treatment, and the integration of properly trained personnel to help clients better understand and improve the behavior and welfare of their pets. Learning, training, and behavior modification should be based on scientifically sound learning principles and an understanding of the normal behavior of the species. These tools, combined with evidence-based medicine, should help practitioners develop a sound treatment protocol, rather than using domination and punishment to change behavior, neither of which is helpful for the owner or the pet.

Several articles in this issue will help the general practitioner feel more comfortable with behavioral medicine. Drs. Seibert and Landsberg begin by helping veterinarians put behavioral medicine into an internal medicine paradigm. Handling behavior problems in practice and using auxiliary personnel, including technicians and trainers, is covered well by Shaw and Donaldson, with commentary by Dr. Landsberg. This article also addresses preventive care

0195-5616/08/$ – see front matter
doi:10.1016/j.cvsm.2008.06.001

through early socialization and puppy classes and guidelines on the selection of trainers. Proper trainers can guide owners using positive training and sound science, rather than some of the misguided and heavy handed approaches that continue to be propagated in the popular press and damage the trust between owner and their pet, and ultimately perhaps the human-animal bond. The article by Dr. Seksel provides further detail into how preventive programs can be implemented in the practice for new puppies and kittens. These articles also provide a range of additional resources for the practitioner.

Aggression is an ongoing problem in dogs and cats, and it is dangerous to people and other animals. Examining aggressive animals presents a challenge to clinicians, and Dr. Moffat offers practical and useful solutions for making veterinary visits less stressful for clinicians, owners, and their pets. Management tools that allow veterinarians to give owners immediate help are presented, and Dr. Horwitz outlines how veterinarians can offer these in a practical way to clients. We also hope to further enlighten veterinarians with a new look at owner directed aggression; the article by Drs. Luescher and Reisner help practitioners understand this vexing problem. Dr. Haug tackles the serious problem of canine aggression toward unfamiliar people and dogs and provides practical suggestions on causes and management of this dangerous problem.

Anxiety issues are prevalent in behavioral medicine in dogs and cats. An update on separation anxiety and noise sensitivities, by Drs. Simpson and Mills, will provide veterinarians with an evidence based approach to treatment for owners who continue to struggle with these anxiety conditions. Feline anxiety issues are covered by Dr. Levine, and feline aggression toward people is detailed by Dr. Curtis.

Family dynamics have changed over the past 25 years, and it has become increasingly more common to add new pets to the household, combine two households that both have pets, or introduce new humans into the home whether it is a new baby, new spouse or integrating entire families. Drs. Bergman and Gaskins provide timely and pertinent advice so veterinarians can counsel owners on how to make the new introductions into the home a smooth transition.

Finally, obtaining a pet has taken on new dimensions, with shelters and rescue centers altering the way dogs are acquired and raising questions on selecting and placing dogs into homes. Dr. Duxbury offers current insights into choosing a puppy, and Dr. Marder discusses adoptions from a shelter environment.

In our careers as veterinary behaviorists, we have not only counseled pet owners on how to work with their pet's undesirable behavior, but we have also tried to encourage veterinary practitioners to embrace behavior as an important component of clinical practice through our lectures, workshops, and publications. Along the way, we hope that we have succeeded in helping veterinary practitioners and staff members improve their skills and add more behavior services to their practices. With this in mind, we hope that this volume of

Veterinary Clinics of North America: Small Animal Practice will provide veterinarians with new and useful information in the field of veterinary behavior that can be implemented in each veterinary practice, and perhaps inspire a few more veterinarians to consider the field of veterinary behavior as a specialty area they might wish to pursue. Interested veterinarians should join the American Veterinary Society of Animal Behavior (www.avsabonline.org) or the European Society of Veterinary Clinical Ethology (www.esvce.org); interested technicians should join the Society of Veterinary Behavioral Technicians (www.svbt.org); and those who have an interest in board certification should visit the websites of the American College of Veterinary Behaviorists (www.dacvb.org) or the European College of Veterinary Behavioral Medicine (www.ecvbm.org) to find more details.

We thank all our authors for their hard work and our colleagues, who have offered information in this format before, because they inspired us to contribute to this body of work. John Vassallo, Editor, and his staff at Elsevier, have been instrumental in making these volumes a reality, and their hard work and dedication is much appreciated.

Gary M. Landsberg, DVM
Doncaster Animal Clinic
99 Henderson Avenue
Thornhill, Ontario L3T 2K9, Canada

E-mail address: gmlandvm@aol.com

Debra F. Horwitz, DVM
Veterinary Behavior Consultations
11469 Olive Boulevard #254
St. Louis, MO 63141-7108, USA

E-mail address: debhdvm@aol.com

Vet Clin Small Anim 38 (2008) 937–950

VETERINARY CLINICS
SMALL ANIMAL PRACTICE

Diagnosis and Management of Patients Presenting with Behavior Problems

Lynne M. Seibert, DVM, PhD[a],*,
Gary M. Landsberg, DVM[b,c]

[a]Veterinary Behavior Consultants, 11415 NE 128th Street, Suite 10, Kirkland, WA 98034, USA
[b]North Toronto Animal Clinic, 99 Henderson Avenue, Thornhill, ON L3T 2K9, Canada
[c]Doncaster Animal Clinic, 99 Henderson Avenue, Thornhill, Ontario L3T 2K9, Canada

BEHAVIORAL WELLNESS AND PROBLEM PREVENTION

There is a recognized connection between mental and physical health in the field of human medicine, and this connection is beginning to be recognized in the veterinary field [1]. Chronic stress or anxiety can contribute to physical problems, and, likewise, acute and chronic physical problems can cause or contribute to anxiety-related issues (see the article by Dr. Levine found elsewhere in this issue). In caring for their patients, veterinarians must be attentive to both the mental and physical well being of the patient. Physical well being is not the only relevant feature of a healthy patient. Veterinarians also must address the possibility of mental suffering in their patients and provide relief for these patients with the same compassion that they treat physical ailments.

In addition to treating behavior conditions, prevention should be part of a behavior wellness program. Hetts and colleagues [2] have outlined the important aspects of developing a behavior wellness program in general practices. Veterinary practices need to incorporate owner education that creates realistic expectations and provide counseling about pet selection, assistance with socialization and preventive care, staff education in behavior and humane handling techniques, and timely referral to behavior specialists when indicated.

McMillan and Rollin [3] have expressed concern for the veterinary profession's lack of involvement in addressing concerns related to mental wellness in animals and the importance of incorporating a holistic approach to health that includes both physical and mental well being. A survey of veterinarians in small animal practices in the United States indicates that many practitioners do not feel confident addressing or treating behavior problems in their patients [4]. Only 25% of veterinarians regularly inquired about pet behavioral issues with their clients.

*Corresponding author. E-mail address: ocddoc@msn.com (L.M. Seibert).

0195-5616/08/$ – see front matter
doi:10.1016/j.cvsm.2008.04.001

In a survey of veterinarians in private small animal practices, the following skills were considered important [5]:

Recognizing communication signals and properly restraining patients
Advising owners about early pet socialization
Safely restraining aggressive patients
Knowing how animals learn and how to shape behavior humanely
Obtaining a complete behavioral history
Diagnosing and treating inappropriate elimination and aggression problems in cats
Recognizing and treating noise phobia and separation anxiety in dogs

When veterinarians in small animal practices were asked which skills are most important for a new veterinary school graduate, knowledge about animal behavior ranked sixteenth on the list of important skills. Managing behavior during veterinary visits and safely handling difficult patients is a critical skill. An understanding of behavioral signaling and learning theory assists veterinarians and veterinary staff in minimizing any negative consequences during veterinary hospital visits and helps ensure that future visits can proceed smoothly and without excessive stress [6]. Staff education is important to avoid any situations in which patient welfare, mental or physical, is compromised.

There perhaps is no greater threat to the human–companion animal bond than behavior problems [7]. Behavior problems can result in relinquishment to shelters, abandonment, or euthanasia if mismanaged or left untreated. An estimated 224,000 dogs and cats are euthanized each year in veterinary hospitals as a result of behavior problems [4]. A significant proportion of the millions of dogs and cats relinquished to animal shelters are adult pets with behavior problems [8]. The article by Drs. Marder and Duxbury found elsewhere in this issue discusses pet selection. Inappropriate elimination is a common reason given for relinquishment of both dogs and cats to shelters. In a case-control study, Patronek and colleagues [9] identified significant risk factors for relinquishment of cats to shelters, which included daily or weekly inappropriate elimination. In a survey of owners of cats that engaged in vertical urine marking, 26% of those surveyed did not contact their veterinarians about the problem because many believed that the veterinarian could not help with the problem, and 93% of owners reported consulting with nonveterinary sources instead of, or in addition to, their veterinarian [10].

According to one survey of animal shelters across the United States, approximately 10% of dogs are relinquished because of aggression problems, and nearly 70% of these have bitten at least one person [11]. Early veterinary intervention, active efforts to identify and address behavior issues, and client education about pet behavior would decrease the number of companion animal deaths each year, but only 25% of dog owners reported receiving routine behavioral advice from their veterinarian [12].

BEHAVIORAL MEDICINE IN VETERINARY PRACTICE

Companion animals may be presented to practitioners with a variety of behavioral complaints, including aggression, anxiety, destructive behavior, inappropriate elimination, disobedience, repetitive or compulsive behaviors, and cognitive dysfunction [13]. It is important to determine if the behavior is a normal behavioral response, a response that is normal given the context but is problematic for the owner, an abnormal behavior, or an indication of a primary medical condition. Mills [14] believes that behavior problems derive from (1) actions that have adaptive value for the animal but are unacceptable to the owner, (2) maladaptive responses to environmental stressors, or (3) actions resulting from nervous system malfunction and encourages treatment approaches that focus on the functional value of the behavior and its underlying mechanisms.

For any animal experiencing a change in behavior, the veterinarian should be involved in evaluating the patient's overall health before assuming that the animal needs training or behavior modification. A change in behavior often is the first sign of a primary medical condition. For this reason, it is critical that veterinarians understand normal behavior and recognize when a patient's behavior is abnormal, taking into consideration the patient's age, breed, gender, neuter status, and social environment. Physical illness can cause irritability or aggressiveness, loss of impulse control, changes in house-training capabilities, changes in social interactions, and confusion, and even can contribute to hierarchy disputes in multipet households. Any condition causing pain may decrease a pet's tolerance of handling, reprimands, children, and physical activity. Physical changes resulting in sensory impairment, such as loss or decline in visual capacity, hearing, or olfaction, ultimately will alter the pet's behavior. Central nervous system disorders and endocrine abnormalities also may become apparent from a behavior change rather than another obvious physical symptom.

CLINICAL APPROACH FOR BEHAVIOR CASES

The veterinarian's role in assessing patients that present with behavior symptoms is to evaluate the patient's physical health, obtain medical, nutritional, and behavioral histories, and determine whether the behavior is normal, abnormal, a manifestation of a medical condition, or a combination of these factors. In fact, because behavioral signs can be the first indication of an underlying health problem or a welfare issue, a component of patient evaluation at each visit should include questioning the owners either interactively or through the use of a questionnaire as to whether there are any behavioral complaints or changes since the previous visit. This information is particularly important in assessing older pets, in which sensory decline, pain, tumors, and degenerative diseases including cognitive dysfunction become increasingly common and may be manifested solely as behavioral signs. Abrupt onset of behavioral changes—even aggression—in an older animal should prompt the clinician to ask "Why now?" and to undertake a good medical evaluation.

The minimum database for any patient presenting with behavior symptoms should include a medical history, behavioral history, complete blood cell count, chemistry panel, and urinalysis. These tests are important in assessing the health of any patient and provide baseline data should psychoactive agents be prescribed. Additional diagnostic tests may be indicated depending on the presenting complaint(s), age of the patient, breed, and medical history.

A thorough behavioral history is critical for an accurate diagnosis. It should include descriptions of the patient's early history, interactions with family members and other animals, housing conditions, and details about the current behavior problems. Pet owners need to be asked for specific descriptions of actual behaviors, including body postures and facial expressions, rather than subjective assessments about the pet's motivation or intentions in performing a given behavior. The behavior history should include a chronologic description of the behavior problem or problems, including an objective description of the behavior, duration, location, eliciting stimuli or circumstances, individuals involved, any attempted interventions or treatments, and the outcomes or responses to interventions. Information provided by the owner about the pet's behavior in the home environment should be combined with direct observations of the patient's interactions with family members and strangers, postural signaling, responses to novel stimuli, and response to behavior modification. Provocative challenges that intentionally induce anxiety or aggression are not necessary for obtaining a diagnosis and may be dangerous. Observations of subtle postural changes and behavioral responses should provide the information necessary for a diagnosis.

Because behavior problems contribute to significant mortality and suffering in veterinary patients, it is important that the veterinarian approach any behavior problem with the same systematic approach used for a medical case, obtaining all the information necessary for a diagnosis and developing a treatment plan that is appropriate for the specific diagnosis. Aggression (growling, snarling, barking, or biting) can be a symptom of a variety of disorders, including encephalitis, portosystemic shunt, resource guarding, fear, osteoarthritis, territoriality, or learned behavior. Prescribing a drug, or any other treatment without a specific diagnosis is unlikely to be successful and may even be dangerous. A study of veterinary diagnostic and treatment approaches for urine marking in cats revealed that 31% of veterinarians did not use historical information regarding deposition of urine on vertical surfaces as a diagnostic criterion for marking [10]. Information about the orientation, location, and quantity of urine deposited is critical in differentiating marking from inappropriate elimination, two different conditions that require different treatment approaches. Improving opportunities for behavior education for veterinarians should begin to address this lack of knowledge about diagnosis of behavioral illness.

MEDICAL DIFFERENTIALS FOR BEHAVIOR SIGNS

Reviews of medical conditions that have been associated with behavioral symptoms are available and include viral diseases, endocrine disorders, neoplasia, toxins, trauma, congenital lesions, infectious agents, degenerative disorders, and allergies [15–17]. Historically, the veterinary profession has focused on differentiating between medical and behavioral conditions, first diagnosing and treating any medical conditions and then attempting to address behavior issues once all medical treatment options have been exhausted. A paradigm shift is needed so that practitioners begin to address medical and behavioral components concurrently to achieve maximum health and wellness for patients. The following example illustrates the importance of a holistic approach to feline house-soiling problems.

Cats that have feline lower urinary tract disease commonly present for inappropriate elimination outside the litter box. It is common for the behavioral symptom of house soiling to persist long after the medical evidence of urinary tract inflammation has subsided. Practitioners who have an understanding of normal litter box behavior and applied learning theory are better able to address the behavioral and physical needs of these patients. Following any illness that results in pain associated with elimination (cystitis, constipation, gastroenteritis), learned aversions to the litter box, the litter substrate, or the litter box location can develop because of classical conditioning. Learned aversions resulting from medical conditions may manifest as house-soiling behavior or lack of burying behavior in litter substrate and may persist after medical symptoms have resolved [18,19]. Environmental or behavioral interventions will be necessary to resolve these problems, in addition to appropriate medical therapies and dietary modifications, and some patients may benefit from anxiolytic medication.

Similar issues can arise in patients presented for aggression when a painful medical condition is present. A dog with otitis externa who experiences painful handling or petting near the infected ear by a family member can develop learned fear reactions to particular individuals. An initial pain-induced aggressive response can persist as fear-induced aggression even after the infection has resolved. In addition, even after the problem has been resolved, the pet may not be aware that further handling no longer leads to pain. Thorough behavioral and medical histories will assist in determining the origin of the behavior and the appropriate course of therapy.

Thyroid Function

A relationship between hyperthyroidism and aggression in cats has been suggested, although a direct causative relationship has not been proven. It is possible that aggression and hyperthyroidism occur in cats as comorbid conditions [16]. Likewise, a relationship between hypothyroidism and aggression in dogs has been suggested, but no strong support exists for a causative relationship. A controlled study found that there is no significant difference in the values in an eight-analyte thyroid panel for normal (nonaggressive dogs) and aggressive dogs [20]. Evaluating the effects of thyroid supplementation on behavior without the benefit of a control group does not offer any definitive proof of a causative relationship between hypothyroidism and behavioral abnormalities. Thyroid supplementation is likely to cause some changes in behavior even in euthyroid patients, and thus behavior changes in association with thyroid supplementation should not be interpreted as evidence of disease. Although thyroid supplementation, either alone or in combination with other therapies, has been used in the treatment of behavioral conditions in human patients, caution should be exercised before considering thyroid supplementation in canine patients without confirmation of thyroid disease. Only canine patients that have clinical signs of thyroid disease and laboratory evidence of thyroid disease (based on logical test choices and results of total thyroxine, free thyroxine, triiodothyronine, thyrotropin, and/or antithyroid antibodies) should be given supplementation [21].

Behavioral Dermatology

There is a strong relationship between grooming, dermatologic conditions, and anxiety in both humans and pets, and any patient that presents for overgrooming should be evaluated for anxiety-related conditions, with attention to the presence of environmental stressors. Conditions have been categorized as psychophysiologic disorders (primary dermatologic conditions that are influenced by emotional stress), primary behavioral disorders (primary problem is behavioral, and secondary skin manifestations are self-inflicted), secondary behavioral disorders (dermatologic conditions that affect normal behavioral function, social function, or emotional reactivity), or cutaneous sensory disorders (conditions for which the patient experiences sensory discomfort in the absence of an identifiable medical condition) [22]. Thorough diagnostic testing is indicated to address the medical needs of the patient. Underlying medical conditions were identified in 76% of cats presented for presumed psychogenic alopecia, and multiple medical conditions were identified in 68% of these cats [23]. The results of this study indicate that cats presented for self-induced alopecia should be evaluated for food sensitivities, atopy, flea allergic dermatitis, parasitic dermatosis, and bacterial dermatitis. Testing may involve skin scrapings, fungal cultures, skin biopsy, flea control, and hypoallergenic diet trials.

Primary dermatologic conditions are uncomfortable and probably will result in increased anxiety or irritability if chronic. In a survey of dog owners in a general veterinary caseload, a history of a pruritic or malodorous skin disorder requiring veterinary treatment was identified as a statistically significant risk factor for aggressive biting behavior in adult dogs [24].

Although some self-inflicted dermatologic lesions respond to traditional medical therapies, other cases show no obvious medical etiology and require the clinician to consider behavioral origins and therapies. Conditions that may require behavioral interventions include canine acral lick dermatitis, psychogenic alopecia (overgrooming), flank sucking, and feline hyperesthesia syndrome [25]. The behavioral motivation for overgrooming, barbering, or self-injurious behavior is unknown but may involve neurotransmitter changes, environmental stressors, genetic predispositions, concurrent medical issues, or learned conditioning [25,26].

Cognitive Dysfunction

Because disease states are increasingly likely to arise with age, when behavioral changes are observed in the senior pet, medical problems (as discussed previously) should be a primary consideration. A behavioral history also is essential, however, because environmental change and stressors also could account for the behavioral signs. A further complication is that older pets may be less able to adapt to change.

Age-related degenerative changes in the brain can lead to a variety of behavioral signs, commonly referred to as "cognitive dysfunction syndrome." Traditionally these signs have been described by the acronym "DISHA," which refers to disorientation, interactions (or alterations in social interactions with people or other pets), sleep-wake cycle changes, house soiling and deficits in other learned behaviors, and activity (which could be a decrease in activity or an increase in activity including repetitive behaviors and aimless wandering) [27–30]. These signs are not the only signs that can be associated with brain aging, however; deficits in learning and memory are most likely to be the first sign of cognitive decline in both dogs and humans. Because deficits in learning and memory are difficult to quantify clinically in pets, the clinical signs of cognitive dysfunction in dogs commonly are reported to arise at age 11 years or older, whereas laboratory studies indicate that dogs begin to show impairment in memory tasks as early as 6 years of age, [27,29,31]. Learning and memory have been measured objectively and standardized by neuropsychologic testing in the laboratory environment using food hidden under food wells. (For more details, review Refs. [29,31,32].)

Agitation or anxiety are signs associated with frontotemporal dementia and Alzheimer's disease in humans that similarly may be associated with cognitive dysfunction in dogs and cats [33–35]. In fact, as reported in a presentation at the American Veterinary Medical Association in 2006, a search of the Veterinary Information Network message boards found that fear and anxiety, including hypervigilance and vocalization, were the most common behavioral complaints for dogs aged 9 to 17 years (n = 50), followed by separation anxiety, nighttime restlessness, disorientation, wandering and pacing, noise phobias, and compulsive licking [36]. Before a behavioral diagnosis was made, the medical conditions that were considered included cerebral diseases, hypertension, sensory decline, arthritis, pituitary-dependent hyperadrenocorticism, renal and hepatic disease, and the effects of drugs such as prednisone and phenylpropanolamine. In 100 cats aged 11 to 22 years, the most common complaint was vocalization, followed by nighttime restlessness, inappropriate elimination, disorientation, wandering or pacing, anxiety, irritable aggression, fear and hiding, and increased attachment to/dependency on owners [36]. In cats a much wider range of possible medical causes had to be ruled out, including pain (arthritis, dental), hyperthyroidism, renal and hepatic disease, hypertension, concurrent drug therapy, sensory decline, and forebrain diseases [36].

Changes that have been identified in the brains of aging dogs and cats include reduced brain mass, increased ventricular size, meningeal calcification, demyelination, glial changes, a reduction in neurons, neuroaxonal degeneration, an increase in apoptotic bodies, lipofuscin, and beta-amyloid, and increased markers of oxidative stress [37–39]. Studies indicate that both the extent of oxidative damage and the amyloid load correlate with the severity of dysfunction [40–42].

TREATMENT MODALITIES FOR BEHAVIOR DISORDERS

Along with diagnosing and treating concurrent or causative medical issues, the veterinarian should determine the most appropriate treatment options to address the behavior problems. Treatment probably will include owner education, behavior modification focused on relaxation, gradual desensitization, and developing coping skills, environmental modifications that reduce the frequency of inappropriate behaviors and increase the frequency of acceptable behaviors, and, in some cases, pharmacologic interventions. Owner education often requires the practitioner to correct misunderstandings about animal behavior that are prevalent in popular culture and literature and to set realistic expectations for behavioral changes (see the article by Dr. Horowitz elsewhere in this issue).

Behavior modification programs should be based on the specific behavioral diagnoses, unique family dynamics, special needs of the patient and owner, and safety considerations. Programs are based on scientific knowledge of learning theory, motivation, communication, and natural species behaviors. A variety of behavior modification techniques are available for the treatment of behavior problems [43–45]. Many behavior problems need to be managed as chronic conditions. Some problems require lifelong behavior modification and/or environmental management. Regular follow-up is necessary for continued success in managing many of these cases. In a study of fear-related canine aggression cases [46], clinician-initiated, scheduled follow-up appointments resulted in higher satisfaction and reports of positive outcomes by clients than unstructured, owner-initiated follow-up.

Group or private dog training may not be appropriate for every patient and may be counterproductive or even detrimental in patients that have anxiety disorders or aggression problems. The experience and expertise of any individual should be considered before referring any patient for treatment. Anxiety is not a training issue but rather is a behavioral pathology or an aberrant reaction to environmental conditions that responds best to a combination of anxiolytic medication, adjustments to the environment, and exercises targeted at teaching relaxation and systematic desensitization. Referral of aggressive patients presents a potential for liability for the referring veterinarian when the veterinarian refers a client to a nonveterinary consultant. Like anxiety, aggression rarely results from a lack of obedience training. Basic obedience training is unlikely to address the treatment needs of an aggressive patient adequately, and the risk of human injury is great when these cases are mismanaged. Individuals with advanced training in behavioral diagnoses and learning theory from reputable doctoral or masters programs or board-certified veterinary behaviorists can provide appropriate instruction for these patients.

The American College of Veterinary Behaviorists (ACVB), recognized since 1993, currently has 46 board-certified diplomates. These individuals have proven knowledge in the following areas:

Learning theory
Neurophysiology
Neurology
Behavioral pharmacology
Behavioral physiology
General medicine
Diagnostic techniques
Normal behavior of domestic, food animal, laboratory, exotic, and zoo species
Behavioral genetics
Sociobiology
Animal welfare
Research methodology

In most states, only licensed veterinarians legally can establish diagnoses, recommend specific treatment interventions, and prescribe necessary medications. More details about the ACVB and its members are available at www.dacvb.org.

EFFECTIVE USE OF PSYCHOACTIVE AGENTS

Psychoactive medications cross the blood–brain barrier, influence nervous system functions, and produce changes in behavior or motivation. Pharmacotherapy for behavior disorders can ease emotional suffering and manifestations of anxiety, facilitate effective behavior modification, and promote owner compliance by hastening treatment outcomes. The following questions should be considered before prescribing any psychoactive agents [47–50]:

1. Has a complete behavioral history been obtained?
2. Have appropriate diagnostic tests been completed to determine underlying or contributing medical conditions and to provide pretreatment baseline laboratory values?
3. Has a diagnosis or a list of reasonable differential diagnoses been established based on the behavioral history and diagnostic testing? A diagnosis is not the same as a clinical sign. For example, spinning or tail chasing is a clinical sign. A list of differential diagnoses for this symptom might include compulsive disorder, anxiety-induced displacement behavior, partial motor seizure, or attention-seeking conditioned response.
4. Has a behavior therapy program been initiated by the veterinarian? Drug therapy rarely is appropriate as a sole treatment but rather should be used as adjunctive therapy. Patients that have behavior problems must have their environmental and social needs addressed, and a plan for teaching coping skills and addressing the underlying cause of the problem must be developed.

5. Will the potential benefits of the medication outweigh the potential risks? All medications have the potential for side effects. The choice of medication should be based on minimizing the potential for complications by considering the individual patient, pre-existing medical conditions, drug interactions, safety margins, and the practitioner's comfort with the particular medication. The potential for adverse events should be discussed with the pet owner.

6. Does the patient need medication, or will the medication improve the patient's quality of life? The need for pharmaceutical intervention depends on many factors. If a behavior modification program can be accomplished without the use of drugs, or if the stimuli or stressors that elicit the problematic behavior can be avoided, drug therapy might be unnecessary. The frequency of the behavior and the extent that the behavior interferes with normal functioning should be considered also.

7. Is the choice of medication appropriate for the diagnosis? There must be a specific rationale for use of the drug, and the medication use must be appropriate under current standards of practice. This field is advancing rapidly , so it is critical that veterinarians remain current and consult specialists when indicated. The decision to choose a drug or natural supplement should be informed by sufficient evidence-based medical data showing that the use of a particular drug is warranted.

8. Have realistic expectations been set for the effects of the medication? Some therapies require a month or more of treatment before significant progress is apparent. Most drug therapies require concurrent behavior modification programs. Clients must understand the limitations of drug therapy, and veterinarians can improve results through regular progress checks. Veterinarians should strive to help clients understand the difference between improvement and resolution of the problem behavior.

9. For drugs not approved by the Food and Drug Administration and extra-label uses of drugs, has the client been informed about extra-label use? Most use of medication for behavioral disorders in veterinary medicine is extra-label, with the exception of fluoxetine (Reconcile, Lilly Companion Animal Health, Indianapolis, Indiana) for the treatment of separation anxiety in dogs, selegiline (Anipryl, Pfizer Animal Health, Exton, Pennsylvania) for the treatment of cognitive dysfunction in dogs, and clomipramine (Clomicalm, Novartis Animal Health, Greensboro, North Carolina) for the treatment of separation anxiety in dogs. The Animal Medicinal Drug Use Clarification Act of 1994 allows extra-label use of medications if certain conditions are met [47,50]. Extra-label use of medications is acceptable when a valid veterinarian–client/patient relationship exists, the veterinarian has established a diagnosis and the need for medication, which means appropriate and adequate medical and behavioral evaluation have been obtained to justify the diagnosis, prescription records are kept, and the drug used has a specific and accepted rationale. Samples of informed consent statements for extra-label medication use are available [50,51].

10. What is the long-term treatment plan? The veterinarian should outline the expected course of treatment, expected onset of efficacy, and a plan for discontinuing or weaning off of the medication once the behavior problem has stabilized.

11. These same questions should be asked when considering the use of natural therapeutics. Reviewing the evidence for efficacy and safety is essential, because

many herbs and natural supplements have little or no data to support their use, may have the potential for toxicity and side effects, and may be contraindicated with certain health problems or when used concurrently with other medications. Some studies have shown the potential for efficacy of dietary therapy with Canine B/D (Hills Pet Nutrition, Topeka, KS) and with supplements with phosphatidylserine, docosahexaenoic acid, antioxidants, mitochondrial cofactors, and S-adenosylmethionine for cognitive dysfunction in dogs [32,52]. Pheromones also may be useful with a minimum of side effects for the treatment of some behavioral problems associated with anxiety in dogs and cats [53–58]. Other natural ingredients that might be considered for the treatment of anxiety-based conditions on limited initial testing include alpha-casozepine [59,60], l-theanine [61,62], and aromatherapy [63].

TREATMENT FAILURES

Treatment failures can result from owner noncompliance, lack of an effective behavior modification plan, lack of control over environmental factors, lack of response to the medication, or tolerance. Tolerance is a diminished response to repeated administration of a drug. Tolerance can occur as a result of enzyme induction by the liver (pharmacokinetic tolerance) or receptor adaptation and down-regulation (pharmacodynamic or cellular tolerance).

When treatment failure occurs, the veterinarian should review the behavior modification plan and assess owner compliance before switching or augmenting the medication therapy. In the event of an actual treatment failure, switching to another medication often is an effective strategy. If one drug does not work, another might. Even medications within the same drug class sometimes have very different effects in individual patients. Combination medication therapies also can be considered [64]. Before using combination therapies, one should consider any contraindications for their combined use, the potential for increased side effects, and the underlying mechanisms and logic for using the two agents together.

SUMMARY

Behavior problems in companion animals are common and can result in serious and life-threatening consequences unless appropriate treatments are initiated. Veterinarians can use their knowledge and diagnostic expertise to manage both the physical and emotional needs of their patients. Understanding normal behavior is critical in recognizing medical conditions and behavioral disorders and for providing preventive care. A variety of treatment options, including behavior modification, adjunctive medical therapy, psychoactive medications, and alternative therapies, are available for managing behavior problems. A holistic approach to health that recognizes the interconnections between mental and physical well being is essential.

References

[1] McMillan FD. Stress, distress, and emotion: distinctions and implications for mental well-being. In: McMillan FD, editor. Mental health and well-being in animals. Ames (IA): Blackwell; 2005. p. 93–111.

[2] Hetts S, Heinke ML, Estep DQ. Behavior wellness concepts for general veterinary practice. J Am Vet Med Assoc 2004;225(4):506–13.

[3] McMillan FD, Rollin BE. The presence of mind: on reunifying the animal mind and body. J Am Vet Med Assoc 2001;218(11):1723–7.

[4] Patronek GJ, Dodman NH. Attitudes, procedures, and delivery of behavior services by veterinarians in small animal practice. J Am Vet Med Assoc 1999;215(11):1606–11.

[5] Greenfield CL, Johnson AL, Schaeffer DJ. Frequency of use of various procedures, skills, and areas of knowledge among veterinarians in private small animal exclusive or predominant practice and proficiency expected of new veterinary school graduates. J Am Vet Med Assoc 2004;224(11):1780–7.

[6] McMillan FD. Compassionate animal care in veterinary practice. Part II. Expectations and goal setting. Veterinary Technician 1996;17:259–65.

[7] Houpt KA, Honig SU, Reisner IR. Breaking the human-companion animal bond. J Am Vet Med Assoc 1996;208(10):1653–9.

[8] Scarlett JM, Salman MD, New JG, et al. The role of veterinary practitioners in reducing dog and cat relinquishments and euthanasias. J Am Vet Med Assoc 2002;220(3):306–11.

[9] Patronek GJ, Glickman LT, Beck AM, et al. Risk factors for relinquishment of cats to an animal shelter. J Am Vet Med Assoc 1996;209(3):582–8.

[10] Bergman L, Hart BL, Bain M, et al. Evaluation of urine marking by cats as a model for understanding veterinary diagnostic and treatment approaches and client attitudes. J Am Vet Med Assoc 2002;221(9):1282–6.

[11] Salman MD, New JG, Scarlett JM, et al. Human and animal factors related to the relinquishment of dogs and cats in 12 selected animal shelters in the United States. J Appl Anim Welf Sci 1998;1(3):207–26.

[12] Patronek GJ, Glickman LT, Beck AM, et al. Risk factors for the relinquishment of dogs to an animal shelter. J Am Vet Med Assoc 1996;209(3):572–81.

[13] Horwitz DF. Differences and similarities between behavioral and internal medicine. J Am Vet Med Assoc 2000;217(9):1372–6.

[14] Mills DS. Medical paradigms for the study of problem behaviour: a critical review. Appl Anim Behav Sci 2003;81:265–77.

[15] Aronson LP. Systemic causes of aggression and their treatment. In: Dodman NH, Shuster L, editors. Psychopharmacology of animal behavior disorders. Malden (MA): Blackwell Science; 1998. p. 64–102.

[16] Overall KL. Medical differentials with potential behavioral manifestations. Vet Clin North Am Small Anim Pract 2003;33:213–29.

[17] Reisner I. The pathophysiologic basis of behavior problems. Vet Clin North Am Small Anim Pract 1991;21:207–24.

[18] Sung W, Crowell-Davis SL. Elimination behavior patterns of domestic cats (Felis catus) with and without elimination behavior problems. Am J Vet Res 2006;67(9):1500–4, 19.

[19] Horwitz D. Behavioral and environmental factors associated with elimination behavior problems in cats: a retrospective study. Appl Anim Behav Sci 1997;52:129–37.

[20] Radosta-Huntley LA, Shofer FS, Reisner IR. Comparison of thyroid values in aggressive and non-aggressive dogs. American College of Veterinary Behaviorists and the American Veterinary Society of Animal Behavior Scientific Paper and Poster Session. Honolulu (HI);2006. p.15–16.

[21] Ferguson DC. Testing for hypothyroidism in dogs. Vet Clin North Am Small Anim Pract 2007;37(4):647–69.

[22] Virga V. Behavioral dermatology. Vet Clin North Am Small Anim Pract 2003;33:231–51.

[23] Waisglass SE, Landsberg GM, Yager JA, et al. Underlying medical conditions in cats with presumptive psychogenic alopecia. J Am Vet Med Assoc 2006;228(11):1705–9.

[24] Guy NC, Luescher UA, Dohoo SE, et al. Risk factors for dog bites to owners in a general veterinary caseload. Appl Anim Behav Sci 2001;74:29–42.

[25] Luescher AU. Diagnosis and management of compulsive disorders in dogs and cats. Vet Clin North Am Small Anim Pract 2003;33:253–67.

[26] Willemse T, Spruijt BM. Preliminary evidence for dopaminergic involvement in stress-induced excessive grooming in cats. Neurosci Res Commun 1995;17:203–8.

[27] Nielson JC, Hart BL, Cliff KD, et al. Prevalence of behavioral changes associated with age-related cognitive impairment in dogs. J Am Vet Med Assoc 2001;218:1787–91.

[28] Moffat K, Landsberg G. An investigation into the prevalence of clinical signs of cognitive dysfunction syndrome (CDS) in cats [abstract]. J Am Anim Hosp Assoc 2003;39:512.

[29] Landsberg G, Araujo JA. Geriatric behavior problems. Vet Clin North Am Small Anim Pract 2005;35:675–98.

[30] Siwak CT, Tapp PD, Zicker SC, et al. Locomotor activity rhythms in dogs with age and cognitive status. Behav Neurosci 2003;117:813–24.

[31] Studzinski CM, Christie L-A, Araujo JA, et al. Visuospatial function in the Beagle dog: an early marker of cognitive decline in a model of human cognitive aging and dementia. Neurobiol Learn Mem 2006;86:197–204.

[32] Milgram NW, Zicker SC, Head E, et al. Dietary enrichment counteracts age-associated cognitive dysfunction in canines. Neurobiol Aging 2002;23:737–45.

[33] Porter VR, Buxton WG, Fairbanks LA, et al. Frequency and characteristics of anxiety among patients with Alzheimer's disease and related dementias. J Neuropsychiatry Clin Neurosci 2003;15:180–6.

[34] Senanarong V, Cummings JL, Fairbanks L, et al. Agitation in Alzheimer's disease is a manifestation of frontal lobe dysfunction. Dement Geriatr Cogn Disord 2004;17:14–20.

[35] Landsberg GM. The most common behavior problems in older dogs. Vet Med 1995;90(Suppl):16–24.

[36] Landsberg GM. Senior pet anxiety disorders. Honolulu (HI): American Veterinary Medical Association Conference Notes; 2006.

[37] Borras D, Ferrer I, Pumarola M. Age related changes in the brain of the dog. Vet Pathol 1999;36:202–11.

[38] Cummings BJ, Satou T, Head E, et al. Diffuse plaques contain c-terminal AB42 and not AB40: evidence from cats and dogs. Neurobiol Aging 1996;17:4653–9.

[39] Head E, Moffat K, Das P, et al. Beta-amyloid deposition and tau phosphorylation in clinically characterized aged cats. Neurobiol Aging 2005;26:749–63.

[40] Cummings BJ, Head E, Afagh AJ, et al. B-amyloid accumulation correlates with cognitive dysfunction in the aged canine. Neurobiol Learn Mem 1996;66:11–23.

[41] Colle M-A, Hauw J-J, Crespau F, et al. Vascular and parenchymal beta-amyloid deposition in the aging dog: correlation with behavior. Neurobiol Aging 2000;21:695–704.

[42] Rofina JE, Singh K, Skoumalova-Vesela A, et al. Histochemical accumulation of oxidative damage products is associated with Alzheimer-like pathology in the canine. Amyloid J Protein Folding Disord 2004;11:90–100.

[43] Crowell-Davis SL. How dogs learn: the role of rewards and punishment. In: Ackerman L, Landsberg G, Hunthausen W, editors. Dog behavior and training: veterinary advice for owners. Neptune (NJ): TFH Publications; 1996. p. 57–69.

[44] Mills DS. Using learning theory in animal behavior therapy practice. Vet Clin North Am Small Anim Pract 1997;27(3):617–35.

[45] Wright JC, Reid PJ, Rozier Z. Treatment of emotional distress and disorders—nonpharmacologic methods. In: McMillan FD, editor. Mental health and well-being in animals. Ames (IA): Blackwell; 2005. p. 145–57.

[46] Radosta-Huntley L, Shofer F, Reisner I. Comparison of 42 cases of canine fear-related aggression with structured clinician initiated follow-up and 25 cases with unstructured client initiated follow-up. Appl Anim Behav Sci 2007;105:330–41.

[47] Crowell-Davis SL. Introduction. In: Crowell-Davis SL, Murray T, editors. Veterinary psychopharmacology. Ames (IA): Blackwell; 2006. p. 3–24.

[48] Marder AR, Posage JM. Treatment of emotional distress and disorders—pharmacologic methods. In: McMillan FD, editor. Mental health and well-being in animals. Ames (IA): Blackwell; 2005. p. 159–66.

[49] Overall KL. Pharmacological treatment in behavioural medicine: the importance of neuro-chemistry, molecular biology, and mechanistic hypothesis. Vet J 2001;162:9–23.

[50] Overall KL. Pharmacologic treatments for behavior problems. Vet Clin North Am Small Anim Pract 1997;27(3):637–65.

[51] Landsberg G. Informed consent for behavior-modifying drug use. In: Landsberg G, Hunthausen W, Ackerman L, editors. Handbook of behavior problems of the dog and cat. 2nd edition. Philadelphia: Saunders; 2003. p. 518.

[52] Landsberg GM. Therapeutic agents for the treatment of cognitive dysfunction in dogs. Prog Neuropsychopharmacol Biol Psychiatry 2005;29:471–9.

[53] Ogata N, Takeuchi Y. Clinical trial of a feline pheromone analogue for feline urine marking. J Vet Med Sci 2001;63:157–61.

[54] Cerissa A, Griffith CA, Steigerwald ES, et al. Effects of a synthetic facial pheromone on behavior of cats. J Am Vet Med Assoc 2000;217:1154–6.

[55] Mills DS, Ramos D, Estelles MG, et al. A triple blind placebo-controlled investigation into the assessment of the effect of dog appeasing pheromone (DAP) on anxiety related behaviour of problem dogs in the veterinary clinic. Appl Anim Behav Sci 2006;98:114–26.

[56] Tod E, Brander D, Wran N. Efficacy of a dog appeasing pheromone in reducing stress and fear related behaviour in shelter dogs. Appl Anim Behav Sci 2005;93:295–308.

[57] Levine ED, Ramos D, Mills DS. A prospective study of two self help CD based desensitization and counter-conditioning programmes with the use of dog appeasing pheromone for the treatment of firework fears in dogs (canis familiaris). Appl Anim Behav Sci 2007;105: 311–29.

[58] Estelles MG, Mills DS. Signs of travel-related problems in dogs and their response to treatment with dog-appeasing pheromone. Vet Rec 2006;159:140–8.

[59] Beata C, Beaumont-Graff E, Coll V, et al. Effect of alpha-casozepine (Zylkene) on anxiety in cats. Journal of Veterinary Behaviour: Clinical Applications and Research 2007;2:40–6.

[60] Beata C, Beaumont-Graff E, Diaz C, et al. Comparison of the effect of alpha-casozepine (Zylkene) versus selegiline hydrochloride on anxiety disorders in dogs. Journal of Veterinary Behaviour: Clinical Applications and Research 2007;2:175–83.

[61] Berteselli GV, Michelazzi M. Use of l-theanine tablets (Anixitame™) and behavior modification for treatment of phobias in dogs: a preliminary study. In: Landsberg G, Matiello S, Mills D, editors. Proceedings of the Sixth IVBM/ECVBM-CA. Brescia (Italy): Fondazione iniziative Zooprofilattiche e Zootechniche; 2007. p. 185–6.

[62] Dramard V, Kern L, Hofmans J. Clinical efficacy of l-theanine tablets to reduce anxiety-related emotional disorders in cats: a pilot open-label clinical trial. In: Landsberg G, Matiello S, Mills D, et al, editors. Proceedings of the sixth IVBM/ECVBM-CA. Brescia (Italy): Fondazione iniziative Zooprofilattiche e Zootechniche; 2007. p. 114–5.

[63] Wells DL. Aromatherapy for travel-induced excitement in dogs. J Am Vet Med Assoc 2006;229:964–7.

[64] Simpson BS, Papich MG. Pharmacologic management in veterinary behavioral medicine. Vet Clin North Am Small Anim Pract 2003;33:365–404.

ELSEVIER
SAUNDERS

Vet Clin Small Anim 38 (2008) 951–969

VETERINARY CLINICS
SMALL ANIMAL PRACTICE

Handling Behavior Problems in the Practice Setting

Gary M. Landsberg, DVM[a,b,*], Julie Shaw, AS, RVT[c],
Jean Donaldson, BSc, CPDT[d]

[a]North Toronto Animal Clinic, 99 Henderson Avenue, Thornhill, ON L3T 2K9, Canada
[b]Doncaster Animal Clinic, 99 Henderson Avenue, Thornhill, Ontario L3T 2K9, Canada
[c]Animal Behavior Clinic, Purdue University, 625 Harrison Street, West Lafayette, IN 47907, USA
[d]The San Francisco Society for the Prevention of Cruelty to Animals,
The Academy for Dog Trainers, 2500 16th Street, San Francisco, CA 94103, USA

THE VETERINARY CLINIC AND BEHAVIOR PROBLEMS

The veterinary clinic plays a critical and primary role in the prevention and treatment of behavior problems. Studies have shown that some of the principle risk factors for relinquishment include insufficient advice at the first few puppy visits, insufficient guidance and reading material for cat owners, and unrealistic expectations by the owners [1,2]. These deficits can lead to pet relinquishment; on the other hand, counseling pet owners on normal behavior and the prevention of behavior problems is likely to strengthen the pet–owner bond. Although many behavior problems are, in fact, normal behaviors that require advice and management, some problems may require medical diagnostics (a much more detailed consultation to make a diagnosis) to determine the prognosis and to develop appropriate treatment strategies, which might include drug therapy. Therefore the veterinarian, behavioral technician, veterinary staff, and trainers all play important roles in preventing and treating behavior problems to provide the most appropriate level of care for each case (see the article by Horwitz elsewhere in this issue for management suggestions for behavior problems).

THE ROLE OF THE VETERINARIAN

It is the veterinarian's responsibility to develop the hospital's policy for the treatment of behavior problems. The veterinarian also is responsible for ruling out health issues and diagnosing behavior problems, because the treatment of behavior problems is considered practicing veterinary medicine, and the Model Practice Act states that only a veterinarian can diagnose disease. The first step, therefore, is to assess the patient's behavioral signs and its physical health to

*Corresponding author. E-mail address: gmlandvm@aol.com (G.M. Landsberg).

determine whether the behavior is normal, abnormal, a result of a medical condition, or some combination of these factors.

When the behavior is determined to be normal but undesirable for the owners or the household, advice or guidance can be given by a sufficiently educated member of the staff team or by referring the client to appropriate resource material. A technician with training in behavior can be a valuable resource in providing appropriate preventive advice and in assisting the veterinarian in behavioral screening and in the diagnosis and treatment of behavior problems. The role of the technician (Box 1) and how technicians can be effectively used in the practice are discussed in a later section of this article.

Often dogs can benefit greatly from the hands-on guidance of a trainer. Veterinarians should understand the important role that trainers serve in

---

Box 1: Role of a behavior technician

- Teaching appropriate behavior
- Consulting on the use of training aids
- Conducting puppy classes
- Conducting obedience training, service dog training, companion dog training
- Correcting training problems
- Dealing with normal but undesirable behavior such as jumping up or attention-getting behaviors
- Training to accept restraint, grooming, and veterinary procedures
- Prevention of behavior problems
- Using behavior modification for problem behavior in specific situations (eg, using response substitution to remedy aggression between two specific dogs in obedience class; desensitizing a dog to a specific object or situation it fears)
- Using behavior modification for behavior disorders under veterinary supervision
- Giving advice on managing animals that have behavior problems until a consultation is performed
- Taking a clinical behavioral history
- Designing a behavior modification program within the framework of a prescribed treatment plan
- Case follow-up, monitoring side effects of drug treatment

NOT: making a diagnosis

NOT: prescribing drugs

NOT: treating behavior disorders (eg, aggression of a dog towards other dogs in general or generalized fear or anxiety) unless instructed or supervised by a veterinarian

Data from Luescher AU, Flannigan G, Mertens P. The role and responsibilities of behavior technicians in behavioral treatment and therapy. Journal of Veterinary Behavior: Clinical Applications and Research 2007;2:23–5.

helping prevent behavior problems and in managing undesirable behavior (Box 2). As discussed later, however, the client is well served only if appropriate trainers are recommended.

When the pet's undesirable behavior has been shaped by previous experiences (ie, learning and consequences) and there are no abnormal or medical components to the problem, the owners require the guidance of a trained behavioral professional which might be (1) a behavioral technician or staff member under the guidance of the veterinarian, (2) a veterinary behaviorist, or (3) an applied animal behaviorist. Many canine cases also may benefit from or require the additional guidance of a trainer who can demonstrate the use of the techniques that the owner will need to use to change the behavior of the patient.

When the behavior is determined to be abnormal or there is a medical component to the behavior, the veterinarian must create and prescribe the treatment plan including the management procedures, behavior modification techniques, and medications to be used. At this point if the practitioner does not feel sufficiently trained in diagnosis or treatment of the problem that has

---

Box 2: Role of dog trainers

- Teaching appropriate behavior
- Consulting on the use of training aids
- Conducting puppy classes
- Conducting obedience training, service dog training, companion dog training
- Correcting training problems
- Dealing with normal but undesirable behavior such as jumping up or attention-getting behaviors
- Training to accept restraint, grooming, and veterinary procedures
- Prevention of behavior problems
- Using behavior modification for problem behavior in specific situations (eg, using response substitution to remedy aggression between two specific dogs in obedience class; desensitizing a dog to a specific object or situation it is afraid of)
- Using behavior modification for behavior disorders under veterinary supervision

NOT: treating behavior disorders (eg, aggression of a dog to other dogs in general; generalized fear or anxiety) unless instructed or supervised by a veterinarian

NOT: making a diagnosis

NOT: drug treatment

Data from Leuscher AU, Flannigan G, Mertens P. The role and limitations of trainers in behavior treatment and therapy. Journal of Veterinary Behavior: Clinical Applications and Research 2007;2:26–7.

been presented, the most suitable option might be to refer the case to a board-certified veterinary behaviorist. Alternately the veterinarian may seek the guidance of a veterinary behaviorist or work together with an applied animal behaviorist for a combined program of medical and behavioral guidance. It is the veterinarian's duty, however, to give the clients a prognosis and to modify the prescribed treatment plan during follow-up care. Implementation of the program also may require some personal guidance from a veterinary behavioral technician or trainer who is familiar with the tools and behavior modification techniques that have been recommended.

For further details on the veterinarian's role in diagnosing and managing patients that have behavior problems, please refer to the article in this issue by Seibert and Landsberg.

The veterinary behavioral technician can be a valuable resource for providing and overseeing the behavioral services offered in the veterinary clinic. The behavioral technician can play a primary role in clinic's preventive counseling program, in the demonstration and sale of behavior management products, in setting up puppy kindergarten and kitten kindergarten programs, and in screening each client to identify any emerging behavioral problems. In addition, a behavioral technician can play an important role in a behavior consultation before, during, and after the consultation. The Society of Veterinary Behavioral Technicians (svbt.org) is a useful resource for educating and increasing the awareness of behavior as an important veterinary service.

Preventive Counseling

Each clinic should be involved actively in preventive counseling so that each new pet owner receives sufficient education to provide for the behavioral needs of the pet and to understand the basics of reward-based training. The role of managing the preventive counseling services can fall under the direction of the behavioral technician. At each visit the veterinary clinic should provide behavioral guidance, support material in the form of handouts, reading lists, and websites, and the names of trainers whom the clinic recommends. The behavior technician might help coordinate the entire staff team to use the time and expertise of each staff member better and to ensure consistent and complete behavioral guidance. When behavior problems arise because the owners do not have a sound understanding of normal behavior and learning principles, or when the owners have inappropriate expectations for their newly obtained pet, some time can be set aside after the veterinary visit to meet with the technician for behavioral guidance. Depending on the problem, however, it might be more prudent to schedule a separate visit to focus on the specific issues, to provide support material, and to demonstrate techniques and products that might be appropriate or necessary. Enrichment devices (eg, feeding and chew toys), products for odor control (eg, for indoor elimination problems), and devices for improved control and training (eg, body harnesses, head halters, clickers, targets, remote reward systems) are items that might be worthwhile stocking and selling in the clinic.

Another way to disseminate effectively information about normal behavior and about how pets learn and to provide a controlled environment for socialization and early training is for veterinary clinics to provide puppy or kitty kindergarten classes. One study found that the combination of puppy class attendance and the use of a head halter was associated with a reduction in relinquishment [3]. Therefore, if the clinic has appropriate and sufficient space on premises or some other readily available space nearby, the veterinary technician can be instrumental in the implementation of puppy or kitten kindergarten classes. Adult training classes, agility classes, and private consultations also might be offered, depending on the expertise of the behavioral technician and the clinic staff team. It also might be possible to combine efforts with a local trainer to assist in offering these classes to client's pets.

Guidelines for Setting up a Puppy Kindergarten

A puppy kindergarten class should be directed toward puppies between the ages of 7 and 16 weeks of age. The primary goal of a kindergarten program is to teach owners how to socialize their puppy properly. Owner education should include assisting the owner in developing fair and realistic expectations for the puppy. The correct use of reward-based training programs and the potential side effects of aversive or punishment-based training methods should be discussed. It also is helpful to teach the owner common canine body language, including signs of stress and conflict. The owners can be shown techniques to decrease a stressful situation and how to apply simple behavior modification techniques to socialize the puppy properly to the stimulus. High-risk puppies or puppies with concerning behavior can be identified for early intervention, which may include a behavior consultation with the veterinarian.

Specific topics in the curriculum should include

- Housetraining issues
- Teaching bite inhibition
- Body-handling techniques for future grooming and medicating
- Destructive behaviors
- Preventing guarding issues
- Preventing separation anxiety
- Discussing puppies and children safety
- Beginning clicker training techniques
- Teaching "sit," "down," "come," and walking on a loose leash
- Teaching desensitization and response substitution techniques

Sample lessons from the Purdue ABC Puppy Course are given in Box 3.

Pets with Behavior Problems—The Technician's Role

It often is the role of the veterinary technician to create client awareness when dealing with behavior problems. A veterinary technician can educate the client in treatment possibilities and set a positive foundation for the behavior consultation. Often clients do not understand that there are viable and successful treatment options, which may include pharmacologic treatment and behavior

Box 3: Curriculum: ABC puppy school

Wheels and sounds

Review

- Crate training
- Housetraining

Problem prevention

- Ringing a bell to go outside
- Bite inhibition
- Preventing guarding of food/objects

Teach

- "Take it," "drop it"
- "Sit"
- "Leave it"

Homework

Bite inhibition: *Start Me Up* (gray book), p. 29

Food bowl safety: *Prevent* (red book), pp. 6–13

Trading: *Prevent* (red book), pp. 14–15

Drop it, take it, leave it: *Games* (orange book), pp. 8–11

Sit: *Jr. Obedience* (blue book), pp. 18–19

Next week: bring a puppy ready to discover obstacles!

Obstacles

Review

- Ring a bell
- Bite inhibition
- Guarding

Problem prevention

- Child proofing/rough handling
- Which hand? "Shake"
- Jumping

Teach

- On/off, in/out
- Wait at the door
- "Down"
- Stand

Homework

Child proofing: *Prevent* (red book), pp. 1–5

Which hand?: *Games* (orange book), pp. 30–33

Jumping up: *Prevent* (red book), pp. 20–23

On/off, in/out: *Prevent* (red book), pp. 16–19

Down and stand: *Jr. Obedience* (blue book), pp. 20–23

Next week: wear a costume, uniform, or article of clothing such as a hat, sunglasses, or other scary" piece of clothing

(*continued on next page*)

Costumes

Review

- Child proofing
- Jumping

Problem prevention

- Destructive behavior
- Retrieve
- Scary monster
- "Gotcha" collar grab

Teach

- "Come" (recall)
- Hide and seek, round robin, out of the gate

Homework

Retrieve: *Games* (orange book), pp. 22–25
Scary monster: *Prevent* (red book), pp. 29–31
Come (recall): *Jr. Obedience* (blue book), pp. 24–30
Hide and seek: *Games* (orange book), pp. 14–18
Round robin: *Games* (orange book), pp. 26–29
Out of the gate: *Games* (orange book), pp. 28–29
Introduction to collar and leash: *Jr. Obedience* (blue book), pp. 10–11

Next week: bring a puppy ready to visit the veterinary hospital

Health and handling

Review

- Destructive behavior
- Retrieve
- Scary monster
- "Gotcha" collar grab

Problem prevention

- Alone training
- Handling
- Daily walks

Teach

- Walking on a loose leash

Homework

Time alone: *Prevent* (red book), pp. 32–33
Handling: *Prevent* (red book), pp. 24–28
Loose leash: *Jr. Obedience* (blue book), pp. 10–17
Follow me: *Games* (orange book), pp. 19–21

Next week: bring objects and toys that move and make noise

Puppies can begin the program at any class.
Courtesy of Purdue University Animal Behavior Clinic, West Lafayette, Indiana; with permission. Text: The ultimate puppy kit. Available at: www.premier.com.

modification. One of the best ways to make clients aware that behavior problems can be addressed and treated is to question each client at each visit as to whether the pet has any behavior issues. This questioning might be accomplished by using a behavior and health questionnaire provided and completed in advance of the visit. At the very least, questions about behavioral health should be part of the history-taking process by either the veterinary technician or veterinarian at the start of each visit. The behavioral history might begin with a nonspecific question, such as, "Is there anything you'd like to change about your pet's behavior?" If the owner is uncertain or cannot list specific concerns, it might be more prudent, to ensure that nothing is overlooked, to go through a list of more direct questions such as, "Does your pet show any unwanted responses when visitors come to your home?" or "Does your cat use the litter box consistently and regularly?" The behavioral history should be a critical component of each veterinary visit, because behavioral signs might indicate an emerging medical or behavioral disease process. In addition, it demonstrates to the client the clinic's interest in knowing about any behavioral issues. Depending on the presenting complaint, the behavioral technician, in consultation with the veterinarian, can take a triage approach, classifying the problem as one that requires veterinary assessment, one in which the technician can ensure that the client has the appropriate advice, resources, and guidance to deal with the problem, or one for which the owner should seek out an appropriate trainer.

Triage—When Should the Veterinarian See the Pet?

During the history taking the technician should determine whether the client might be dealing with a behavior disorder with or without concurrent medical issues, whether the issues are related specifically to lack of training or inappropriate owner expectations, or whether the situation calls for intervention to prevent a problem.

Because veterinary technicians and support staff cannot diagnose behavior problems, it is crucial for the technician to determine whether the situation is still in the preventative stages. Clarifying which issues and situations are important, creating a consistent protocol for dealing with them, and discussing the results with the entire staff allow better implementation.

The following case examples are presented for consideration.

A 12-week-old puppy is reported by the owners to be "dominant"
This description by the owner gives the technician little information except to indicate the owner's need for further education. The technician should ask, "What is the puppy doing that makes you feel he is "dominant?" The client may reply that the puppy is jumping on the children and "biting" them.

At this point, preventive guidance and information and resources on play biting can be provided, and puppy classes could be recommended so the technician or trainer can evaluate further whether the puppy is demonstrating normal puppy behavior that can addressed in the puppy class setting or atypical behavior that should be addressed by the veterinarian.

A client complains that the dog barks all day

The technician should get specific information about when the dog is barking and whether there is a stimulus for the barking. If the dog is barking while the owners are home and available, and the eliciting stimulus are the squirrels in the neighbor's yard, this behavior probably does not indicate an anxiety disorder and could be investigated more fully by the veterinary technician. If the client indicates the dog is barking when they leave for work and continues throughout the day, the dog should be scheduled with the veterinarian for a behavior consultation to determine if separation anxiety is a possible diagnosis.

An owner reports a 5-month-old dog is having bowel movements in the house

The technician should determine whether the dog has been examined recently and, if not, a physical examination should be scheduled. If an examination (including a fecal examination) has occurred recently, the technician should determine if the appetite or stools are abnormal in any way. If there are no abnormalities, the next step is to find out whether the puppy ever has been fully housetrained and when the accidents are occurring. If the puppy keeps its crate clean and soils only when the owners are not watching, basic guidance in housetraining should be provided. If the accidents occur only in the dog's crate or only when the owner leaves the house, however, a video camera could be set up to determine the dog's anxiety level during those times. After reviewing the video, the veterinarian and technician can determine if a behavior consultation is in order.

The Role of the Veterinary Technician During a Behavior Consultation

A veterinary technician can educate the client in treatment possibilities and set a positive foundation for the behavior consultation. Often clients do not understand that there are viable and successful treatment options, which may include pharmacologic treatment and behavior modification.

A first step is to help the client prepare for the consultation by recommending a practical and effective management plan until the appointment to prevent the client from becoming injured from an aggressive pet and to prevent the pet from learning from bad experiences (ie, clients should stop all punishment) or from performance of the ongoing behavior. Examples include avoiding any situation that triggers aggression or, in the case of a dog with possible separation anxiety, placing the dog in day care until the appointment (see the article by Horwitz found elsewhere in this issue for a more detailed discussion of the management of behavior problems).

Evaluation of the current status and stability of the human–animal bond can help the technician prioritize appointments. For example, if the clients indicate that they "are at their wit's end and can't take anymore," the situation should be given a high priority and addressed as soon as possible, before the bond is damaged further and the pet isrelinquished.

Helping the client have appropriate expectations for the consultation is essential. The clients should be asked what their goal is after consultation; if they are uncertain, the technician can help them articulate the issue more clearly. For example, if the client says, "We've lost all hope for changing our dog's aggressive behavior toward strange dogs and aren't sure how a behavioral consultation could help," the technician could ask, "If Spot's behavior toward other dogs were improved to your satisfaction, what would that look like?" The client may respond, "We don't expect to be able to take him to a dog park, but we would like to be walk him without fear of his knocking us down in the attempt to attack a dog he sees on the walk." The technician's response might be, "That is a very reasonable expectation, and there are numerous behavior modification techniques the veterinarian may include in your dog's treatment plan to facilitate your goal." If the owner's expectations for improvement exceed what is likely to be practical, however, the technician should help the owners understand that a behavioral assessment can help determine what goals realistically can be achieved so that the owners then can determine if it is practical for them to proceed.

Instructing the client about what to bring to the behavior consultation appointment will help the appointment proceed more smoothly. Because food often is used for motivation and rewards, it is helpful to make sure the patient is hungry when it arrives and that the client supplies the patient's favorite treats. The clients should bring collars, leashes, and other training tools that have been used or presently are being used to help manage the pet. Videotapes can be very useful, and most clients are receptive to bringing videos showing the patient in its normal environment. If multiple pets are involved, a videotape of their interactions both with the owner present and without the owner present should be requested. If the issue is inappropriate elimination, it is helpful to request a diagram of the home with notations depicting windows/doors, locations where stool and urine accidents have occurred, the locations of food and water bowls and litter boxes, and the favorite resting areas of each pet.

Assembling an accurate behavioral history is also a priority. The veterinary technician can acquire the preliminary basic history over the telephone or by mailing the history form and a return envelope to the clients before the appointment. Included in this communication should be information about the fee structure and any cancellation policies.

During the consultation, the veterinarian will need to finish collecting the necessary history, make the diagnosis, and develop a treatment plan. A behavioral technician also can play an important role in the consultation. During the behavior consultation the veterinary technician can determine the patient's trainability and recognize which current control behaviors (eg, "sit," "down," "stay," "come") the patient understands. The technician can explain and demonstrate the treatment options that the veterinarian prescribes, including clicker training, demonstrating to clients how they might teach the behaviors that will be needed during behavior modification exercises (ie, "go to a mat," "down"), desensitizing the pet to a head collar or muzzle, and determining its motivation for various rewards. Sometimes working away from the owner to determine which behaviors have been conditioned inadvertently by the owner can help the technician understand what needs to be explained to the owner. For example, a dog presented for aggression toward strange dogs could be taken for a walk by the veterinary technician to determine the severity and reactivity level of the aggression, the body language demonstrated, and the responsiveness to potential behavior modification techniques.

1. The technician may find the aggression does not occur when the dog is walked without the owner present. This finding may indicate to the veterinarian that there may be strong conditioned component to the behavior and may influence the treatment plan. The veterinary technician's observations of the dog's body language when meeting another dog without the owner present also will assist the veterinarian in determining whether the behavior is defensive or offensive. It often is helpful also to see the dog walked in the owner's presence, to see how the behavior and body language of the dog changes.
2. The veterinary technician can report the degree of the patient's reactivity, including the distance at which the patient reacts to another dog, and can report whether the aggression has the potential of being redirected toward the owner.
3. The veterinary technician also should report on how the patient responded to training tools (eg, a head collar) and behavior modification techniques (eg, counterconditioning and response substitution).

The Role of the Technician Following the Consultation

At the conclusion of the consultation, the technician can demonstrate and teach the prescribed behavior modification techniques, demonstrate training techniques, demonstrate the use of such training tools as a head collar, clarify the treatment plan for the client, and provide any handouts or support material that might be useful.

Specifically the technician should

- Clarify and explain the diagnosis to the client, when appropriate emphasizing that the issue is common and that treatment is available.
- Emphasize that the treatment plan the veterinarian is prescribing should give both the client and the pet relief and that this is only the first step in the treatment. More can be done, and the staff will work closely with them throughout the process.
- Advise the client about any potential side effects of medication.
- Demonstrate prescribed training techniques such as "going to a mat" and "down-stays" and explain to the client that they are teaching and helping the pet develop new and important coping skills.
- Demonstrate and have the owner practice using training tools such as putting on and using a head collar.
- Use the opportunity after the veterinarian has left the consultation to answer questions about the patient's problem or treatment plan. This time can help technicians build rapport with the client that will be beneficial during follow-up care.

Behavior consultation follow-up

Successful treatment of behavior cases can be influenced greatly by follow-up care. The success of follow-up care depends on how well veterinary technicians are used in this aspect of treatment. The veterinary technician can give the client positive feedback, clarify the treatment plan, and answer questions about training and behavior modification techniques. If the owners become frustrated or treatment does not seem effective, the veterinary technician can alert the veterinarian so that changes in the treatment plan can be made.

Methods of follow-up care can include telephone conversations, e-mail communication with the owner, and possibly videotapes of the owner applying the prescribed behavior modification techniques for evaluation. When no progress is being made, return visits may be scheduled.

Technician-Driven Behavior Programs

It may be determined during follow-up care that the client requires more hands-on education. The veterinary technician may make separate behavior modification appointments to assist the owner. Behavior modification training sessions could be conducted in-hospital or in the client's home. The advantage of conducting the sessions in the client's home are that the technician can determine methods for making the techniques fit seamlessly into the client's home and life style. For example, if the dog's aggression in the home is focused around the front door, the veterinarian may have prescribed desensitization to the door opening and also counterconditioning to the doorbell ringing and going to a place away from the door (response substitution) when someone comes to the door. The technician may go to the client's home and demonstrate these techniques to assure the client can apply them in the home environment. These sessions should be scheduled, and a behavioral consultation fee should be assessed.

Conclusion

The success of a hospital's behavior health program can be related directly to how well the technical staff is used in the treatment and prevention of behavior problems. The benefits to the hospital include bonding the client to their pet, bonding the client to the hospital, decreasing veterinarian time needed for the treatment of behavior problems, and making the technician feel valued, well used, and appreciated.

THE ROLE OF DOG TRAINERS

Selecting a Dog Trainer

Dog training is an unlicensed and unregulated profession in the United States and Canada. There currently are no legal constraints on methods in terms of safety or efficacy, and there is no organ of consumer protection. In fact, in certain cases practices that contravene existing anti-cruelty statutes have been non-prosecutable when done in the name of dog training (S. Hetts, personal communication, 2008), because the term "standard industry practice" is expandable to include virtually any technique that has appeared in print at any time (see Table 1).

The Association of Pet Dog Trainers, founded in 1993, puts on an annual educational conference and produces a quarterly newsletter, but professional membership is open to anyone, and there is no credential standard or scientific vetting for either conference presenters or newsletter submissions. The nonmandatory Certified Pet Dog Trainer (CPDT) designation is available to trainers who accumulate a sufficiency of hours teaching classes, training dogs, and coaching dog owners, obtain references from one client, colleague, and veterinarian, and then pass a written examination.

There is no formal educational requirement to be a dog trainer. Three sets of optional guidelines exist for the practice of dog training:

1. The American Humane Association's Guide to Humane Dog Training [4]
2. The Delta Society's Professional Standards for Dog Trainers [5]
3. The Association of Pet Dog Trainer's Code of Professional Conduct and Responsibility [6]

All three emphasize, with varying degrees of detail, that trainers should exhaust well-executed methods based on positive reinforcement of desired behaviors along with behavioral management (antecedent control) before considering the use of aversive stimuli. Thus, although there is some convergence on the principles that ought to govern dog training, it is difficult to assess the degree to which working trainers adhere to them or the degree to which pet dog owners are aware of their existence. It therefore is a "buyer beware" market, often to the detriment of owners and their pets.

Furthermore, the field of dog training has long been under the shadow of the social dominance construct. Loose extrapolations of interpretations of behavior described in captive wolf research have been co-opted by dog trainers since the 1970s to justify the use of coercive and dangerous physical confrontation techniques. Although research in wild-wolf models has diminished the importance attributed to hierarchy models [7], and dog trainers increasingly are accessing and applying the animal learning literature, the notion recently has re-emerged that forcing dogs into submissive postures can serve as a virtual panacea for a wide range of behavior problems, including those that have strong fear components. The popularity of the dominance construct, in spite of the paucity of research supporting its existence in domestic dogs and substantial agreement by clinicians specializing in behavior that techniques derived from animal learning laws are more efficient and carry lower risk of side effects, may result partly from the strong tendency of status-interested humans to project motives and theory of mind capacity to other creatures with which they have strong social bonds [8]. For examples of dog training techniques in the popular printed media that in some cases show a continued reliance on dangerous and inhumane practices, see Table 1.

The following is a suggested list of criteria for clients and other animal professionals to use in assessing a dog trainer's competence and adherence to professional and ethical standards:

1. Basic education, such as a CPDT and bachelor's or graduate-level degree in a relevant discipline such as psychology or education. Continuing education unit credit quotas are necessary to maintain a CPDT designation, but many non-CPDT trainers do attend conferences, seminars, and workshops. Non-CPDT trainers who do so usually include their commitment to continuing education in their promotional materials.

Table 1
Examples of dog-training techniques in the popular printed media showing a continued reliance, in some quarters, on dangerous and inhumane practices

Author(s)	Title	Year First Published	Training Objective	Technique
Most, Konrad	Training Dogs: A Manual	1954	Reduce snarling	Whipping dogs with switch until dog "submits" ("heavy cuts should only be applied to the powerful muscles on the fore- and hindquarters and on the back")
Koehler, William	The Koehler Method of Dog Training	1962	Reduce digging	Hole dug by dog is filled with water and dog's head held under "until he is sure he's drowning," repeating next day whether dog digs or not
Margolis, Matthew and Siegal, Mordecai	Good Dog, Bad Dog	1973	Increase obedience	"Corrective jerk" on choke chain. "The dog may whine or cry out ... Do not be disturbed by this ... More than likely the animal is trying to manipulate you."
Volhard, Joachim and Fisher, Gail	Training Your Dog. The Step-by-Step Manual	1983	Sit/stay	Dog wearing a clip-on choke collar that sits high on the neck (to avoid muscle lower down on neck) is jerked harshly upwards "at the first sign that your dog is thinking about moving"

Author	Book	Year	Topic	Advice
Bauman, Diane	Beyond Basic Dog Training	1986	Coming when called	Untrained dog is placed on leash and abruptly "snapped" toward handler after cue given
Monks of New Skete	The Art of Raising a Puppy	1991	Dominate puppy who "merits it"	"Shake down": both sides of the neck are grabbed, the dog's front end is lifted off the ground, and the dog is shaken several times (more "dominant breeds" should be firmly cuffed under chin)
Benjamin, Carol Lea	Dog Training in Ten Minutes	1997	Walking on leash	After a week of 5- to 10-minute sessions of inducing following with voice or toy, handler walks with dog on leash, changing direction abruptly and unexpectedly so that dog hits the end of the leash ("clotheslining")
Millan, Cesar	Cesar's Way	2006	Preventing threatening dog from attacking	Place an umbrella, walking stick, or anything a person happens to be carrying in front to "look bigger" (this advice also given to children)

2. Use of the standardized language of applied behavior analysis. This use demonstrates acquaintance with the laws governing how animals learn and the ability to access the valuable pure and applied literature on operant and respondent conditioning and to have meaningful exchanges with applied behaviorists and veterinary behaviorists. Clients should be taught to beware of trainers who assert that dog training is in innate talent that cannot be taught or learned, who invent their own terminology, or who disparage "book learning" while claiming that having years of experience is the key or only criterion for the competent practice of dog training.

3. Transparency of motivators employed. Trainers who train without the use of aversive stimuli almost invariably advertise themselves as "all-positive," "force-free," or "dog-friendly." Trainers who employ aversive stimuli either alone or in conjunction with other means typically avoid direct statements about their motivation choices, refer to dogs having an innate "desire to please," and use obfuscating or euphemistic language (such as the term "corrections" or "vibration" for the application of choking or electric shock), frequently involving quasi-mystical or "pack leader" rhetoric. Consumers are advised to inquire directly, "How will my dog be motivated?" Another effective screening question is whether the trainer requires any special type of collar or refuses to use certain training devices such as head collars or harnesses. Trainers requiring choke or prong collars, however they market their approach, inevitably use these devices to dispense punishments. Finally, a client should request the opportunity to witness a training session or a group class before signing up. During a private training session or a group obedience class, there should be timely use of toys, food, praise, and play as reinforcers; there should be clear instructions to owners, and under no circumstances should dogs be jerked by collars, forced into positions, struck with hands or implements, sprayed with water or noxious substances, or have items thrown at them. Owners should be treated respectfully and professionally. The ratio of dogs to instructors and assistants in a group setting should not greatly exceed three or four to one. Written handouts or homework should be given to support the exercises and to prompt owners to practice on their own. If the owner is unable to execute a particular task, the trainer should be able to suggest an alternate training method to help with understanding and learning rather than ascribe blame to either the dog or the owner.

4. Adequate rehearsal, client support, and follow-up in private training. A single consultation with instructions and behavior modification plans subsequently delivered to the client without follow-up sessions is irresponsible practice. Most behavioral problem resolution involves significant investment of time and changes of habit by the client, as well as the development of mechanical training skills. There are almost no adult learners who can make these changes and acquire these skills without supervised step-by-step coaching, repetition of concepts, and continued support.

Board and Train

Some trainers offer a "board and train" service, wherein the dog is housed at the trainer's facility for a period of 2 to 6 weeks to be trained. This service is a valid option for obedience behaviors and certain behavior problems but is inappropriate for problems such as separation anxiety, which actually can be exacerbated by the disruption in access to the owner. Clients considering this option should be made aware by the trainer that there is no outcome guarantee and that the owners still will have the tasks of "transferring" the training to themselves and of maintaining any gains with good practices. There is no option that takes the owner completely "off the hook" vis-a-vis training the dog. It is vitally important in a board and train situation that the trainer's methods be well understood and references be provided, because the training takes place behind closed doors.

Future Trends

A consumer-driven movement to demand licensing of dog trainers, with rudimentary education as prerequisite, would be a significant improvement. For instance, completion of undergraduate-level courses in animal learning and motivation and applied behavior analysis would seem a minimum requirement for someone whose job is to change behavior. Making currently optional practice guidelines mandatory would provide an eventual licensing body a means of evaluating objectively whether breaches of professional conduct have occurred.

SUMMARY

Every veterinary clinic should have sufficient staff and veterinary training and appropriate resources to guide owners in properly understanding, shaping, and managing a pet's behaviors. Common emerging problems in new pets can benefit greatly from early intervention that educates owners about normal behavior and about reinforcing what is desirable in a pet's behavior and provides referral to a trainer who can guide the owners in achieving these behaviors effectively and positively. Therefore, the guidelines within this article are intended to help veterinarians choose trainers in their community to whom they can refer their clients for their basic training needs and to describe the role that trainers can play in helping owners implement the behavior management programs that need to be implemented. Veterinarians and their technical staff must be constantly vigilant and proactive in identifying any behavior changes or behavior problems, because early intervention allows diagnosis and treatment before the problem escalates in intensity, frequency, or severity. At this point the practitioner must decide if there is an organic or medical cause to the problem, and whether the problem is within the scope of the expertise of the veterinarians and technical staff in the clinic. If the case requires further diagnostic evaluation and treatment advice, referral to a veterinary behaviorist might be most prudent. When treatment advice requires that owners improve their level of training and control to implement a behavior modification program effectively, the behavioral technician and the trainer can play critical roles in helping the owners implement the program effectively.

SUGGESTED READINGS

Dog Training and Behavior Modification

Donaldson J. Oh behave! Dogs from Pavlov to Premack to Pinker. Wenatchee (WA): Dogwise Publishing; 2008.

Donaldson J. Perfect Paws in 5 days featuring Jean Donaldson's modern training methods DVD. San Francisco (CA): Perfect Paws Productions; 2007.

Donaldson J, Dunbar I. Fighting dominance in a dog whispering world DVD. Sixes, OR: Dogtec; 2007.

Donaldson J. The culture clash. Berkeley, CA: James and Kenneth Publishers; 2005.

Dunbar I. Sirius dog training DVD. Berkeley, CA: James and Kenneth Publishers; 2006.

Dunbar I. Before and after getting your puppy. Novato, CA: New World Library; 2004.

Dunbar I. How to teach a new dog old tricks. Berkeley, CA: James & Kenneth; 1991.

Miller P. The power of positive dog training. Hoboken, NJ: Howell Book House; 2001.

Pryor K. Don't shoot the dog; the new art of teaching and dog training. Lydney, Gloucestershire: Ringpress Books; 2002.

Reading and Resources for Veterinarians

Client Behavior Handout Series. American Animal Hospital Association. Phildadelphia, PA: Elsevier Saunders.

Bowen J, Heath S. Behaviour problems in small animals—practical advice for the veterinary team. Ames, Iowa: Blackwell Publishing; 2005.

Hart BL, Hart LA, Bain M. Canine and feline behavior therapy. 2nd edition. Denver, CO: Blackwell; 2006.

Hetts Suzanne. Pet Behavior Protocols. American Animal Hospital Association; 1999.

Horwitz DF, Neilson JC. Blackwell's five-minute veterinary consult clinical companion canine and feline behavior. Iowa (IA): Blackwell Publishing; 2007.

Horwitz H, Heath S, Mills D. BSAVA manual of canine and feline behavioral medicine. Gloucester (UK): British Small Animal Veterinary Association; 2003.

Horwitz D, Landsberg GM. Lifelearn CD of client behavior handouts. edition. 2008. Available at: http://www.lifelearn.com/c3/3000a.html. Accessed May 10, 2008.

Journal of Veterinary Behavior – Clinical Applications and Research – Elsevier.

Journal of Applied Animal Behaviour – Elsevier.

Landsberg G, Hunthausen W, Ackerman L. Handbook of behavior problems of the dogs and cat. 2nd edition. London: Elsevier; 2003.

Lane J. Understanding and improving client compliance. Veterinary Technician 2003;24(12): 850–3.

American Veterinary Society of Animal Behavior. Available at: http://www.avsabonline.org. Accessed May 10, 2008.

American College of Veterinary Behaviorists. Available at: http://www.dacvb.org. Accessed May 10, 2008.

Companion Animal Behaviour Therapy Study Group. Available at: http://www.cabtsg.org. Accessed May 10, 2008.

European Society of Veterinary Clinical Ethology. Available at: http://www.esvce.org. Accessed May 10, 2008.

European College of Veterinary Behavioural Medicine Companion Animals. Available at: http://www.ecvbm.org. Accessed May 10, 2008.

Reading and Training Opportunities for Veterinary Technicians

Academy of Veterinary Behavioral Technicians. Available at: http://www.avbt.net. Accessed May 10, 2008.

Association of Pet Dog Trainers. Available at: http://www.apdt.com. Accessed May 10, 2008.

Purdue University's 5 Day DOGS! course. Available at: http://www.vet.purdue.edu/animalbehavior. Accessed May 10, 2008.

The Karen Pryor Academy. Available at: http://www.karenpryoracademy.com. Accessed May 10, 2008.

Society of Veterinary Behavioral Technicians. Available at: http://www.svbt.org. Accessed May 10, 2008.

References

[1] Patronek GJ, et al. Risk factors for relinquishment of cats to an animal shelter. J Am Vet Med Assoc 1996;209:582–8.

[2] Patronek GJ, et al. Risk factors for relinquishment of dogs to an animal shelter. J Am Vet Med Assoc 1996;209(3):572–81.

[3] Duxbury M, Jackson J, Line S, et al. Evaluation of association between retention in the home and attendance at puppy socialization classes. J Am Vet Med Assoc 2003;223(1):61–6.

[4] Ehrhardt J. American Humane Association's guide to humane dog training. Englewood (CO): American Humane Association; 1998–2001.

[5] Hetts S, Miller K, Reid P, et al. Professional standards for dog trainers: effective, humane principles. Bellevue (WA): Delta Society; 2001.

[6] Board of Directors of the Association of Pet Dog Trainers. Code of professional conduct and responsibility. Adopted. Greenville (SC): The Association of Pet Dog Trainers; 2003.

[7] Mech David L. Alpha status, dominance, and division of labor in wolf packs. Available at: http://www.mnforsustain.org/wolf_mech_dominance_alpha_status.htm. Accessed May 9, 2008.

[8] Donaldson Jean. Oh behave! Dogs from Pavlov to Premack to Pinker. Wenatchee (WA): Dogwise Publishing; 2008.

Vet Clin Small Anim 38 (2008) 971–982

VETERINARY CLINICS
SMALL ANIMAL PRACTICE

Preventing Behavior Problems in Puppies and Kittens

Kersti Seksel, BVSc (Hons), MRCVS,
FACVSc (Animal Behaviour), MA (Hons)

Sydney Animal Behaviour Service, 55 Ethel Street, Seaforth, New South Wales 2092, Australia

Pets are an integral part of today's society. Up to 60% of households own pets in various countries around the Western world [1–3]. People keep pets for many reasons including companionship, sport, prestige, and security [4,5]. Owning pets has been shown to benefit owners physically and psychologically. Many pets, however, are surrendered or euthanized each year, and behavior problems are cited as one of the major reasons for the relinquishment of pets [6–9]. The role of the veterinary profession is vitally important in informing current and future pet owners about the behavior of animals.

Animal behavior is a topic of great interest to many in the community, as evidenced by the media attention and the numerous books, articles in popular journals, and television and radio shows devoted to the topic. Unfortunately some of the information available to the pet-owning community and the general public is outdated, misleading, or even detrimental to the welfare of the pet. Therefore it is imperative for veterinarians to provide their clients with up-to-date, practical, and humane information about how to care for their pets that also addresses the welfare of the animals.

BEHAVIOR PROBLEMS

Behavior problems are a major reason for dogs and cats being surrendered to an animal shelter, and several studies have examined these issues.

Dogs that had not attended obedience-training classes were 68.1% more likely to be surrendered. Other risk factors included being sexually intact (30.9%), eliminating inside regularly (19.3%), and not receiving veterinary attention (65.7%) [8]. Dogs were more likely to be surrendered if they exhibited boisterousness (10%), aggression directed toward people (7.7%), and aggression toward other dogs (9%) [7].

Studies also have shown that house soiling is the most common reason for the surrender of cats, followed by problems with other pets and aggressive behaviors [6].

E-mail address: kersti@ava.com.au

0195-5616/08/$ – see front matter
doi:10.1016/j.cvsm.2008.04.003

Dogs and cats were more likely to be relinquished if there was another pet in the household, especially if the other pet had been acquired within the previous year. Dogs acquired from a shelter were at increased risk of being relinquished for behavioral reasons [6].

On the positive side, Duxbury and colleagues [10] found that puppies that attended puppy socialization classes, wore head collars as puppies, responded to basic commands, and were handled frequently as puppies were less likely to be surrendered.

These findings show that the veterinary profession has a major role in decreasing the risk of pets being surrendered or euthanized. From studies of the reasons for pet relinquishment, it is apparent that veterinary advice needs to focus strongly on behavioral issues. Although traditionally the emphasis has been on preventative health care, and this aspect of pet well being should not be minimized, behavioral advice always should be incorporated. The behavioral advice needs to include how to select a suitable pet, the source of the pet, the effects of adding another pet to a household, housetraining, and the importance of socialization and training to dogs and cats.

PREVENTION OF PROBLEMS

To help minimize problematic behaviors and therefore increase the retention rate of pets in the home, the focus should be on three key areas: selection, socialization, and stimulation.

Selection

Selection of a suitable of pet is a critical issue. Informing potential owners about suitable choices for their individual circumstances before they actually acquire a pet would be the ideal situation.

This is a valuable service that veterinarians should offer, but the advice needs to be objective and not influenced by personal biases. Internet services such as "Select - A - Pet" (www.petnet.com.au) also are available to help potential owners choose a pet and consider factors such as the physical and personality characteristics of various breeds, owner lifestyle, owner expectations, and personal preferences (see the article by Duxbury and Marder elsewhere in this issue).

Veterinary advice should include information on where to acquire a pet and its physical characteristics and also on the most suitable age for acquisition, gender, the importance of socialization, and how to house and care for the pet (bedding, feeding, training, exercise, and health care requirements). Further details are given the article by Duxbury and Marder elsewhere in this issue.

Owners should be informed that adding another pet to the household may be problematic, particularly if a dog sourced from a shelter is added to the household [6]. If owners do decide to acquire another pet, advice on how to introduce the pet into the household harmoniously will be important. The use of synthetic pheromone analogues such as dog-appeasement pheromone (DAP, Ceva Santé Animale, La Ballastière, Libourne, Cedex, France) and Feliway (Ceva Santé Animale) has been shown to be useful in helping pets assimilate into the household by minimizing stress. Owners should be advised that for maximum benefit the diffusers should be plugged in about a week before the pet comes into the home and should stay plugged in continuously for the following month. The diffusers should be placed in the area where the puppy or kitten spends most of its time, and the pet should have easy access to the diffuser (ie, be able to lie next to the diffuser should it wish).

The first veterinary visit for puppies and kitten often takes longer than 15 minutes, so ideally at least 30 minutes should be scheduled for this appointment. This visit should cover the physical and psychologic needs of the pet and introduce the owner to the veterinary practice as a lifelong source of advice on behavioral issues.

Socialization

Pets need to be socialized to fit into society. "Socialization" is the term used for the process by which individuals learn and perform behaviors expected of them by society. In the case of dogs and cats, socialization is, therefore, a special learning process in which the puppy or kitten learns also to accept the close proximity of members of its own species as well as members of other species [11]. Lack of socialization, shown by inappropriate responses to people or other animals, is one of the many issues that lead to abandonment of pets [6].

Puppy socialization and training classes ("puppy preschools" and "kitten kindergarten" classes) are one way to socialize puppies and kittens, to expose them to various stimuli in a nonthreatening way, and to teach good manners as expected by the society in which they live [12–14].

Because these classes can help form the basis for the future behavior, it is important that they be conducted in a manner that sets the puppies and kittens up for success and does not overwhelm them with too many stimuli.

It also is important to limit attendance at these classes to puppies and kittens that are still within the period of development defined as the socialization period. Only puppies under 14 weeks of age and kittens under 10 weeks of age should be enrolled in the classes. Owners of older puppies should be encouraged to attended juvenile puppy classes, and owners of older kittens should be encouraged to attend classes but to leave their cats at home.

This age limit is crucial, because dogs and cats that are older interact differently with each other and learn differently. The same is true with children: school classes and sporting teams do not combine 5-year-olds and 15-year-olds. Just because a puppy is small in size (eg, a Chihuahua) does not mean that it is psychologically or physiologically young. Having older puppies in the classes can be damaging to a puppy's development.

For maximum benefit of both the owners and their pets, the classes need to be well thought out and run by experienced people. Conducting them in a veterinary clinic by experienced staff members will help the puppies and kittens, as well as the owners, have positive associations with a veterinary visit.

Having the first class "pet free" allows many behavioral issues to be addressed and attendees to concentrate without the distraction of the cute puppies and kittens. When the puppy or kitten arrives for the next class, some basic material already has been covered.

Giving advice on teaching good manners and on appropriate toys and other tools available to owners will help keep the pet and owner happy. Topics that should be covered in these classes include housetraining, litter box care, use of head collars, physical exercise requirements, mental stimulation environmental enrichment, suitable toys and games, and neutering.

The classes also provide the opportunity to educate owners about the principles of reward and punishment. Although people often talk about reward-based training, punitive methods still are used in many instances. The American Veterinary Society of Animal Behavior recently published guidelines (www.avsabonline.org) on punishment that are worth reviewing with staff and clients. Additionally, many owners also do not have a clear concept of what a reward or punishment is and the effects that rewards and punishments have on the emotional development of their pet and the bond that will develop. Rewarding socially appropriate behaviors and ignoring inappropriate or unacceptable behaviors is a concept that still is unfamiliar to many.

Sample puppy class structure

Also see the article by Landsberg, Shaw, and Donaldson elsewhere in this issue for an alternative puppy class format.

Introductory class. Ideally each class session lasts about 1 hour, and the first class should be puppy free so the owners can concentrate without funny, furry distractions [15]. It allows the participants in the group to meet one other, and the person running the class can give a formal or informal presentation to set the aims or objectives for the classes. This puppy-free class also helps owners discuss problems that they already may be experiencing with their puppies without the distraction of puppies. Additionally, it can be explained to owners that the focus of these classes is not on play but on socialization and teaching good manners.

Explaining to owners that puppies always should be rewarded for appropriate behavior and ignored for inappropriate behaviors is an important part of this first session. It also provides the ideal opportunity to dispel the dominance myth [16] and to help owners understand that being "dominant" or "alpha" is not necessary and indeed can be detrimental to raising a well balanced puppy that is socially acceptable and a pleasure to own.

Handouts covering the common problems that have been discussed (eg, housetraining, mouthing, and chewing) should be distributed.

Class one. In the first class with puppies, the puppies should arrive on lead and stay on lead. Puppies are let off lead only when owners are instructed to do so, and this may not happen in this class or even at all. No more than two puppies should be off lead at any one time. This allows puppies to learn manners when greeting each other rather than just rushing over and expecting to play.

The most important behavior that owners should be taught to put on cue is "settle." Rewarding puppies when they are calm and quiet by using just the owner's whispering (soft) voice rather than food rewards is of major benefit in helping owners manage their dog's behavior.

Other behaviors that are taught in this class are "come" and "sit" using positive reinforcement (food). For example, holding the food above the puppy's nose and slowly moving it up and back over the puppy's head will lead the puppy to start to sit. As soon as the puppy sits, a reward is given. No words are needed until the puppy performs the behavior reliably. Only then is the action paired with the word "sit." At no stage should puppies be forced to sit by pulling up on the lead or be pushed into the "sit" position with pressure on the rump.

Because veterinary examinations include handling of feet, ears, mouth, and body, it is important for puppies to learn early that these activities are non-threatening, and these classes are an ideal opportunity to help the puppies learn to tolerate these examinations. Methods of grooming, giving pills, cleaning teeth, and clipping nails can be demonstrated during the class. Problems such as housetraining, chewing, and biting also should be discussed, and hand-outs should be given to help owners recall this information.

Class two. The puppies should arrive on lead and remain on lead. The owners should be asked to reward the puppies for being calm and quiet. Puppies are asked to demonstrate the behavioral cues ("sit," "come") they were taught at the previous class. In this class, behaviors such as "down" can be put on cue. The class also allows the opportunity to discuss other health issues and to teach more about canine body language and senses.

Class three. Each owner is asked to demonstrate the behaviors that that they have been practicing putting on cue in the previous week. More behaviors such as "stay" and how to walk on a loose lead can be introduced into the puppy's repertoire. The use and usefulness of head collars also can be demonstrated during this class.

Class four. In this final class the owners may "dress up," bringing in "odd" things such as sunglasses, canes, hats, and skateboards, so that the puppies can be exposed to some novel experiences in a nonthreatening manner. Puppies also could be exposed to vacuum cleaners, hairdryers, and brooms so they can learn that such items are not to be feared.

The class may conclude with some games, such as a mock agility course or other types of obstacles. The classes finish with a "graduation" ceremony.

Sample kitten class structure

Introductory class. Each class session should last about 1 hour, and the first class should be kitten free so the owners can concentrate without furry distractions [17]. The kitten-free session allows participants to meet one other, and the person running the class can give a formal or informal presentation to set the objectives for the classes. The class should cover common problem behaviors of cats.

Explaining to owners that kitten always should be rewarded for appropriate behavior and ignored for inappropriate behaviors is an important part of this first session.

Handouts covering the common problems that have been discussed (eg, litter training, biting, and scratching) should be distributed.

Class one. Kittens should arrive in cat carriers or cages and should not be let out until instructed by the person leading the class. In this class owners can be shown how to handle kittens appropriately and how to teach them to relax or settle on cue. Teaching owners how to massage their kittens to relax them should form part of this first class. Kittens can be taught to come and sit on cue using food rewards (tiny, tasty treats such as chicken and cheese are useful).

Class two. In this class owners can be shown how to groom and pill the kitten, trim nails, and check ears. Kittens can be taught to walk on a lead or accept a harness. Many owners need to be taught how to play appropriately with the kitten; part of this discussion should address not using human body parts (hands and fingers) as toys. Having suitable toys for sale is helpful so owners can interact appropriately with their kitten.

The class concludes with a "graduation" ceremony, and handouts that cover the topics discussed should be given.

Stimulation

Although most owners realize that dogs need physical exercise, many do not recognize that cats also need physical exercise. Many owners, however, are not aware of how much mental exercise and stimulation their pet needs.

All animals require an environment that allows them to be physically stimulated (exercised) and mentally stimulated (cognitively and/or emotionally motivated/exercised). This stimulation is especially important for animals that are confined, whether in their own backyard, an apartment, or in a zoo. All animals need to be provided with a complex, stimulating environment that allows them to carry out activities and gives them choices, both physically and psychologically. Confined animals often are understimulated because choices are not available or because the choices are made or enforced for them. When such stimulation is not available, pets may develop problem behaviors (eg, become vocal or destructive) in an attempt to gain attention or look for other stimulation [18,19].

Dogs are a social species and need regular interaction with others, be it with other dogs or with their owners. Dogs are not designed to live alone outside for long periods as their owners' lives get busier. It is important that they live in an environment that is interesting, complex, and stimulating.

Dogs benefit greatly from training, off-lead exercise, agility training, interactive play with owners and other dogs, and toys. Foraging devices can also provide hours of entertainment and exercise the dog's mind as well as its body.

Similarly, cats need to have regular interactions with their owners. Cats can be trained and learn tricks. Many commercial toys for cats are available, but many readily available and inexpensive objects such as ping-pong balls and cardboard boxes can provide hours of entertainment.

Toys need to be changed on a regular, even daily, basis to maintain the pet's interest. Pets need to be taught how to play with the toys, and owners need to be aware of this need for learning. Owners also need to be taught how to interact appropriately with the pet and not to use human body parts as toys. Safety considerations are an essential part of choosing a suitable toy. Toys should be checked regularly so that unsafe toys can be replaced immediately.

Indoor cats have special needs because they are reliant on their owners to provide a stimulating environment. The provision of vertical space with shelves to climb up on and cubbies to hide in is even more important to these cats. Cats need places to hide. Tunnels, paper bags, and cardboard boxes can provide good hiding places, especially if placed up high. It is important in multi-cat households that one cat is not able to corner, trap, or block access to escape from another cat in these hiding places.

Additionally, cats need access to a suitable scratching post to express their normal behavior. An indoor garden box with grass, catnip, or catmint for cats to nibble on and roll in can provide enjoyment for many cats.

Hiding the cat's dry food in a number of places around the house and letting the cat "hunt" for its dinner also can provide physical and mental exercise for cats.

PREVENTABLE PROBLEMS
Housetraining
Eliminating inside is one of the major risk factors for euthanasia or abandonment for both dogs and cats. Advice on housetraining therefore is essential for puppy and kitten owners. For any training to be successful, it is essential to "set up for success" and not allow a puppy or kitten to make a mistake in the first instance.

Puppy housetraining
Puppies need supervision at all times until they learn where they are expected to eliminate. Puppies generally need to eliminate soon after waking up, after meals, or after play. The puppy needs to be taken out to eliminate at these times and also whenever it starts to circle or sniff. When the puppy has urinated or defecated, praise and/or a tasty treat should be given immediately after the event, not when the puppy is back inside the house.

If the puppy does eliminate inside, it is best to ignore the incident. A puppy that is reprimanded when it eliminates in front an owner may associate the punishment with the owner's presence and not with the act of eliminating. The puppy may actively avoid eliminating in the presence of the owner so that it is difficult to praise the puppy for eliminating in the desired location.

Taking the puppy to the same location to eliminate helps the puppy associate this spot as a toileting area. Cueing specific words with the event (eg, "go potty") also can help teach the dog to eliminate on command.

Crate training also may be a useful tool to help housetraining. This topic can be discussed at puppy classes, because it is of great benefit in housetraining as well in preventing destructive behaviors.

Feline litter box training
Cats also can have elimination issues even though many people consider their care to be easy in this aspect. Although most cats easily accept the litter tray as a toileting area, not all do. Owners need to understand that, for a cat to use a litter tray, it needs to be easily accessible, in location as well as size of litter tray. Litter trays need to be cleaned often and placed in areas that allow some privacy. Some cats prefer one tray for urine and another for feces, and some cats do not like to share litter trays. The type of litter used and the depth of the litter also affect the cat's desire to use a litter tray. If the kitten uses an inappropriate location, the owner should be advised to focus immediately on the location and substrate the cat is using and on whether the cat is using the litter for urine, stools, and whether occasionally or not at all. This information provides an opportunity to make immediate adjustments to the box, the litter type, cleaning frequency, or location as well as methods of preventing use of inappropriate areas before the problem develops into a learned aversion or preference.

Growling
Many owners still feel that puppies should not be allowed to growl at them in any circumstances. This attitude is attempts to stop the behavior may be detrimental to the dog. It also potentially puts the owner at more risk later when the dog may no longer give a warning (growl) but just bites.

Growling is a normal part of the canine communication repertoire, and dogs may growl when they are aroused (eg, in play) as well as a warning signal. It is important that owners are taught how to respond appropriately to a growl, because trying to eliminate a growl may lead to escalating aggression [16].

It always is important to look at the context in which the dog growls. If a puppy is growling around its food bowl, there are several ways to manage the problem. One way may be to feed the dog alone and not approach it at all. Another is to teach the dog that having a person approach the dog while it is near the food bowl is a positive experience. This goal may be achieved by giving the dog an almost empty food bowl with food of low value (to the dog) in it. Then, as the dog eats, the owner drops small amounts of more desirable food into the bowl. Finishing this exercise with a high-value treat also can be helpful. This process teaches the puppy that having people near food bowls is a positive experience and also helps build a positive relationship with the owner. Repeating this exercise four or five times a day is important.

A puppy's growling when the owner wants to retrieve an object that has been stolen (eg, a sock) is best approached by ignoring the puppy and not chasing it or turning the process into a game. The puppy can also be taught to "give" on cue, which involves swapping the "stolen" article for something else (eg, a food treat or a toy) that the puppy sees as being more valuable or more exciting.

Mouthing And Biting

Young puppies explore their environment with their mouths, so using their teeth to interact and explore is part of the normal learning process. Chewing is discussed later under destructive behaviors. Some puppies, however, also use their teeth when interacting with their owners, and this biting/mouthing can lead to many problems (including fear of owners and escalated aggression) as owners try to discourage this behavior.

It is important not to use hands (or feet) when trying to discourage a puppy from biting/mouthing. Puppies may interpret these actions as part of a game and increase the intensity and frequency of the biting. Trying to "dominate" the puppy by scruff shaking, rolling it on its side ("alpha roll"), pinning it to the ground until it stops struggling, biting the puppy, growling at the puppy, or using any physical force is unhelpful in teaching the puppy the appropriate or acceptable behavior and can border on being or actually be abusive. These methods are outdated and potentially dangerous and have no place in current veterinary medicine. They do nothing to engender the human–animal bond and do not compromise the welfare of the puppy.

If the puppy does bite or mouth a human body part, the first step is to move away and not allow the puppy any more interaction. The puppy should be taught to "settle" on cue and be rewarded for relaxed behavior. The puppy also should have access to appropriate chew toys to which the owner can direct this behavior. The focus always should be on rewarding appropriate behaviors rather than on punishing unacceptable ones.

Some puppies bite when playing with their owners, usually when the puppy becomes highly aroused. Teaching the puppies to settle on cue is a useful way of managing this behavior, as is stopping play before the puppy gets highly excited. Exercising the puppy's mind and body, as discussed earlier, is also useful in managing this behavior.

Destructive Behaviors

Destructive behaviors include digging, chewing, or scratching. It is normal for young animals to express all of these behaviors as part of their development.

For dogs that enjoy digging, a digging pit of its own can limit the damage that is done to the garden. A child's sand pit is ideal. Filled with loose sand or soil and seeded with buried bones, toys, and other treats, it can encourage digging in this area and can be a source of mental as well as physical stimulation.

Young puppies chew when they are teething, and chewing helps develop jaw strength. Dogs also may chew when they are anxious or distressed, and chewing may be an indication of problems such as separation anxiety. The provision of chew toys and food manipulation toys will help focus the dog's activities on suitable objects. Toys need to be changed regularly to maintain interest and to minimize the dog's desire to destroy potted plants and shoes.

Scratching posts are important for cats. These posts can be bought commercially or built at home from pieces of wood nailed together and covered with carpet. The post needs to be stable (so it does not fall over), and, generally, the larger the better (so the cat can stretch out fully). Some cats prefer to scratch on horizontal surfaces, others on vertical ones, so the posts should allow for both preferences. They also need to be covered in a material that the cat wants to use. Attaching toys on strings can also make these posts more interesting. Spraying the synthetic pheromone analogue Feliway can help attract the cat to the area.

Nuisance Behaviors

Jumping up, pulling on a lead, and vocalizing excessively are behaviors that are problematic for owners. These behaviors may be encouraged inadvertently when the puppy is small and cute and become problems only when the dog is fully grown.

In some cases these behaviors can be managed in the early stages simply by ignoring them or by distracting the dog and then teaching an alternative behavior that is more rewarding for the dog. For example, the owner does not look at, touch, or speak to the dog when it jumps up. The owner only responds to the dog when all four feet are firmly on the ground or the dog is sitting. Making eye contact, pushing the dog down, kneeing him in the chest, pinching his toes, and even saying "no" may encourage the behavior to continue, because the dog has received some attention. Teaching the dog to be calm on cue and to sit on cue are important first steps that can be taught in puppy classes.

Having puppies wear head collars and teaching owners how to fit them properly and how to use them effectively helps teach the dog to walk nicely on a loose lead and helps control problems such as stealing, mouthing, and barking in the owner's presence. Many brands of head collar are available; the key is to find the one that best fits the dog. As the puppy grows, it usually is necessary to buy a new head collar to ensure correct fit. With most head collars, the lead attaches under the dog's chin, but on others lead attaches to the head collar on the back of the neck. Dogs need to be introduced to flat collars and head collars slowly, and puppy classes are an ideal time to introduce these tools to puppies.

Vocalization can be a problem for both dog and cat owners. Dogs bark as a form of communication and may bark when they are excited, fearful, anxious, or want attention. Intermittently rewarding the dog for barking may make the behavior more difficult to modify. For example, allowing a dog is inside the house after it barks to prevent neighbors from complaining rewards barking. When the owners are not home, the dog is not able to access the house, so the reward of coming inside is intermittent, and the barking is likely to become even more persistent.

Although most backyards are adequate for the needs of the human occupants, there often is minimal stimulation for the dog, leading to high levels of arousal. A highly aroused dog may vocalize more and even react with barking to falling leaves and shadows as well as to squirrels, opossums, or cats moving within the dog's environment.

Ideally, all dogs need to learn self control and to be relaxed and calm on cue (settle) as puppies. Puppy classes are an ideal place to introduce these concepts to puppy owners. Because dogs are social animals, they are not happy to be alone for long periods. Providing dogs with physical exercise such as walks and swimming can be useful to tire the dogs so they are less likely to vocalize. Agility classes, off-lead exercise, and training also can help minimize vocalization. Playing interactive games (eg, chasings, hide and seek) also is helpful in alleviating boredom and decreasing barking. Having a regular routine also can be helpful.

SUMMARY

As society's expectations of pets evolve and the demographics of pet ownership changes, the role of the veterinary profession in helping maintain pets in the home environment becomes even more crucial. Because the surrender and abandonment of pets that have behavioral problems continues, the veterinary profession needs to be able to provide sensible and practical advice that educates the community about the behavior of pets.

References

[1] Thorne C. Evolution and domestication. In: Thorne C, editor. The Waltham book of dog and cat behaviour. Oxford (UK): Pergamon Press; 1992.

[2] Dumont G. Telephone survey on attitudes of pet owners and non-pet owners to dogs and cats in Belgian cities. Anthrozoös 1996;9(1):19–24.

[3] Australian Companion Animal Council. Contribution of the pet care industry to the Australian economy. Sydney (Australia): BIS Shrapnel; 2006.

[4] MacCallum M, Beaumont M. A study of our attitudes to cat and dog ownership. Melbourne (Australia): Australia: Petcare Information and Advisory Service; 1992.

[5] Willis MB. Breeding dogs for desirable traits. Journal of Small Animal Practice 1987;28: 965–83.

[6] Salman M, Hutchison J, Ruch-Gaille R, et al. Behavioral reasons for relinquishment of dogs and cats to 12 shelters. Journal of Applied Animal Welfare Science 2000;3(2): 93–106.

[7] Ledger RA, Baxter MR. The development of a validated test to assess the temperament of dogs in a rescue shelter. In: Mills DS, Heath SE, Harrington LJ, editors. Proceedings of the First International Conference on Veterinary Behavioural Medicine. Birmingham (UK): Universities Federation for Animal Welfare; 1997.

[8] Patronek GJ, Glickman LT, Beck AM, et al. Risk factors for relinquishment of dogs to an animal shelter. J Am Vet Med Assoc 1996;209(3):572–81.

[9] Patronek GJ, Glickman LT, Beck AM, et al. Risk factors for relinquishment of cats to an animal shelter. J Am Vet Med Assoc 1996;209(3):582–8.

[10] Duxbury M, Jackson J, Line S, et al. Evaluation of association between retention in the home and attendance at puppy socialization classes. J Am Vet Med Assoc 2003;223(1):61–6.

[11] Beaver B. The veterinarian's encyclopedia of animal behavior. Ames (IA): Iowa State University Press; 1994.

[12] Heath S. Puppies in your practice. Veterinary Practice Nurse 1992;4(3):29–30.

[13] Seksel K. Puppy socialization classes. Vet Clin North Am Small Anim Pract 1997;27(3): 465–77.

[14] Seksel K, Mazurski E, Taylor A. Puppy socialisation programs: short and long term behavioural effects. Journal of Applied Animal Welfare Science 1999;62:335–49.

[15] Seksel K. How to conduct puppy socialization and training classes. Western Veterinary Conference Notes. Las Vegas, Nevada, 2006.

[16] Heath.S. Dispelling the dominance myth. In: World Small Animal Veterinary Association Conference notes. Sydney, Australia, 2007.

[17] Seksel K. Training your cat. Melbourne (Australia): Hyland House Publications ; 2001.

[18] Overall KL. Clinical behavioral medicine for small animals. St. Louis (MO): Mosby; 1997.

[19] Landsberg G, Hunthausen W, Ackerman L. Handbook of behaviour problems of the dog and cat. Oxford (UK): Butterworth-Heinemann; 2003.

Vet Clin Small Anim 38 (2008) 983–1003

VETERINARY CLINICS
SMALL ANIMAL PRACTICE

Addressing Canine and Feline Aggression in the Veterinary Clinic

Kelly Moffat, DVM

VCA Mesa Animal Hospital, 858 N. Country Club, Mesa, AZ 85201, USA

Handling aggressive dogs and cats in the veterinary clinic can be frustrating, time consuming, and injurious for both employee and animal. This article discusses the etiology of the aggressive dog and cat patient and how best to approach these cases. A variety of handling techniques, safety products, and drug therapy are reviewed.

Historically, the handling of the small animal veterinary patient focused little on the welfare of the patient and instead on efficiency for the staff. Some rather physical and harsh types of handling still are used in many clinics. Unfortunately, efficiency is not necessarily safer or in the best interest of the animal. Also, injuries to people and animals are more likely to occur during mishandling and are a liability to the hospital. With the greater development and recognition of the human–animal bond, owners' expectations for all aspects of their pet's care have escalated dramatically. Owners wish to be more involved in the pet's medical care and are cognizant of the compassionate or insensitive care the animal receives from the staff. Handling that induces fear and/or aggression should be avoided at all costs. The veterinary community will benefit if each clinic ensures that its veterinarians and staff understand and recognize basic animal behavior to work best with each patient in a kind, safe, and humane manner.

There is a paucity of information on companion animal handling and restraint in the veterinary field, especially with respect to the problem patient, the underlying motivation for aggression demonstrated by some of these pets, and how to handle these cases effectively and humanely. This article reviews the aggressive dog and cat in the veterinary practice and discusses the most appropriate techniques for approaching these patients for a successful physical examination, diagnostics, and treatment. With better handling, injuries are minimized, the staff and the owners are happier, animal welfare and health are improved, and the animal is less stressed and more amenable to handling on future visits.

E-mail address: drmoffat@cox.net

0195-5616/08/$ – see front matter
doi:10.1016/j.cvsm.2008.04.007

THE AGGRESSIVE PATIENT

Aggression can be defined as any focused and motivated harm directed at another individual [1]. Aggression typically is offensive or defensive in nature, with offensive aggression directly or indirectly motivated by resource control and defensive aggression motivated by danger of harm to the individual [1] It is in the best interests of veterinarians and staff to understand these motivations to prevent or manage aggression more successfully in their hospitals. Although a common misconception, dominance (control of resources) is not the primary reason for aggression in the dog or cat, especially in the hospital setting. Considering the setting, it makes more sense that defensive aggression (fear of danger/harm to oneself) is by far the more common cause. Pain, redirected, maternal, and learned forms of aggression also may be contributing factors for aggression directed towards veterinary staff.

PREVENTION OF FEARFUL AND AGGRESSIVE BEHAVIOR IN THE VETERINARY HOSPITAL

Prevention can begin as soon as the pet enters the clinic by instituting a positive welcoming protocol in which pets are greeted by name and offered favored treats. If there are other dogs or cats that might make the new pet fearful, it might be helpful to separate the animals in the waiting room or to place one of the pets immediately into a separate examining room. During the examination, one should focus on the gentle handling of young patients. Treat bags and toys that can be easily disinfected should be in every room, and one should make the pets visit fun (Fig. 1). Examinations, nail trims, and vaccinations should be made as pleasant as possible and associated with extremely delectable treats. A line of Kong stuffing can be placed on the table so the animal will lick it up while a vaccine is administered, or the owners can offer a handful of tiny treats while the technician and veterinarian give an injection. A few clipped

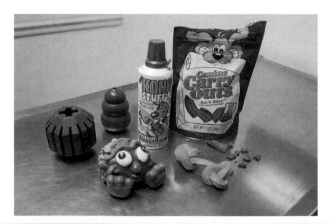

Fig. 1. The hospital should be equipped with treats and toys to offer the pets to distract them while working with them.

toenails can be followed with exuberant verbal praise and treats. Encourage the owners to bring their pets by the clinic for fun visits—visits in which they greet the reception staff, get weighed, and even occasionally are placed in a room where a technician or doctor can come greet them, give them treats, and send them on their way (Fig. 2). These fun visits can be valuable for any pet but are especially important for pets that have shown any fear or anxiety at previous visits. Having the owners fast the puppy prior to the clinic visit, bringing along favorite treats and toys to make the experience enjoyable, ensuring that the owner is positive and gives the pet no reason for increased anxiety, and perhaps even adding a pheromone to the pet's cage or carrier might help overcome any early fears.

EVALUATING THE PATIENT BEFORE APPROACH AND HANDLING

The animal's body language should be evaluated before approaching and handling any patient in the hospital. It is important to notice the ear carriage, the eyes, the position of the lips and mouth, tail carriage, and general body posture. Fear behaviors in both dogs and cats can include lowering and tucking of the tail, leaning backward, crouching or cowering when approached, head held low with eyes averted, piloerection, and flattening of the ears [2,3]. Dogs and cats also may glance in different directions frequently, pant, and stand or sit

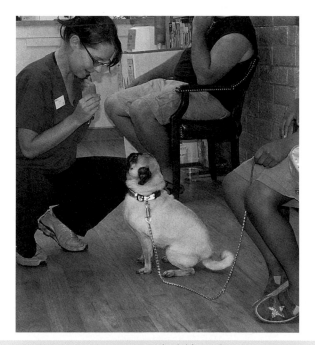

Fig. 2. The receptionist greeting a patient in the lobby with treats.

with one paw raised (Fig. 3) [3]. Although fear may inhibit aggressive behavior as the animal instead freezes or attempts to flee, in the hospital setting the animal usually is prevented from fleeing, and, as the perceived threat increases and escape is prevented, the animal may resort to aggression (fight or flight response) [4]. The dog may begin to threaten actively by growling, lunging, and biting, and the cat may begin hissing, growling, swatting, and biting (Fig. 4). If restrained, the pet may redirect its aggression toward the handler if it cannot gain access to the person who actually is perceived as the threat.

In cases of escalated threats, animals may appear to have a more assertive stance, with ears forward. These animals are demonstrating heightened arousal levels and the most intense defensive behaviors (Fig. 5). Most of the more aggressive behaviors are preceded by other subtle changes as the animal feels more threatened; such changes can include increasing muscle rigidity, closing or tightening of the mouth and lips, and staring [2]. With experience, these animals may learn that use of aggression is successful at removing the stimulus, so that in future encounters the fearful displays may be less noticeable or may arise earlier in the visit (ie, when entering the parking lot or entering the waiting room). Pets that are stressed, anxious, frustrated, or aroused may engage in a displacement behavior [5]. Displacement behaviors may be performed to decrease the animal's arousal or to cope with the conflict the animal is feeling [6]. Displacement behaviors are behaviors that seem to be out of context to the current situation. In dogs, displacement behaviors include yawning, scratching, and smacking and licking of the lips (Fig. 6). In cats, grooming is the most

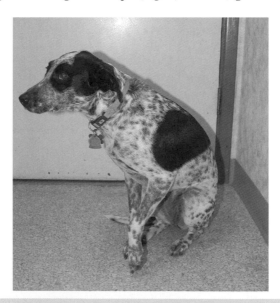

Fig. 3. Fearful dog showing a body posture leaning backward, ears flattened against the head, averted gaze, and paw lifted from the floor. If approached, this dog may freeze or become aggressive.

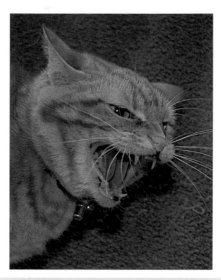

Fig. 4. Defensive/fearful cat demonstrating aggression. The ears are flattened toward the head. The lips are drawn back, and cat is hissing.

common displacement behavior [5]. The staff should monitor the patient for these more subtle anxiety- and fear-based behaviors; if they are seen, extra care should be taken with these patients to avoid escalation to serious and dangerous aggression.

The first and most important recommendation in working with aggressive patients in the veterinary hospital is to slow down! Losing patience with these animals gains nothing and increases the perceived threat. Succeeding on one

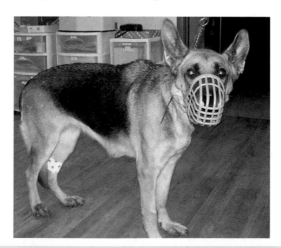

Fig. 5. Fearful dog becoming more highly aroused. The ears are rotating forward, and she is piloerected and is threatening with barking and growling. Note the tucked tail.

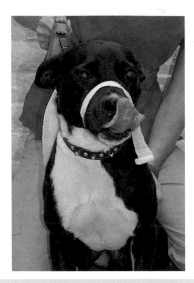

Fig. 6. Displacement behavior: a dog licking its lips/nose while being examined.

visit by using excessive force often leads to a more fearful and difficult second and third visit as the pet makes a negative association to the clinic, staff members, or location (eg, examining table). Second, every staff member should understand basic behavior and body signals. They should be familiar with handling techniques, safety products, and especially their limitations. No staff member should be placed at risk, and appropriate safety precautions (including sedation) should be implemented as needed.

Because nearly all aggression from patients in practice is the result of fear, minimizing stressful situations is paramount for successful handling. Once it is determined that a particular patient is showing fear or displacement behaviors, the staff should give that animal a chance to acclimate to its environment and to the staff's presence. Attempts should be made to examine the patient with the owner present, and the owner should be convinced that the staff is genuinely sensitive to the pet's emotions (and fears). It also is essential that the owner be aware of how to act to help calm the pet and to reduce fear rather than heighten the animal's anxiety. When the owner cannot send the appropriate calming signals, it might be better to separate the pet from the owner to determine if its anxiety is heightened or lessened (as discussed later) and for owner safety.

ENVIRONMENT AND APPROACH

Acquiring a history from the owner while subtly offering the pet patient food treats and/or sitting on the floor to allow the pet to approach are a few methods that can be used when the patient needs additional time to acclimate (Fig. 7). Walking directly to the pet, reaching over it, cornering it, or looking directly

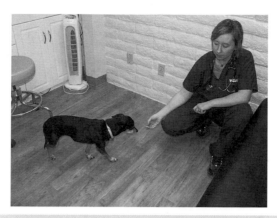

Fig. 7. Technician offering treat while crouching off to the side to encourage dog to approach her.

at it are all confrontational and threatening to the animal and should be avoided (Fig. 8).

When the animal must be examined, kneeling to the side of the dog while softly speaking to it is the preferred approach (Fig. 9). If the pet is already in the hospital ward/cage, opening the door, standing askew, and talking quietly and softly may encourage the pet to approach and will be far less stressful to the pet than reaching into the cage to grab it. Placing smaller dogs and cats on one's lap while performing a physical examination can be more calming and relaxing for them (Fig. 10). Every effort should be made to minimize noise and activities around the pet. Barking dogs, clippers, ultrasonic cleaners, alarms, and the presence of many other employees can be frightening and increase arousal and reactivity of the patient.

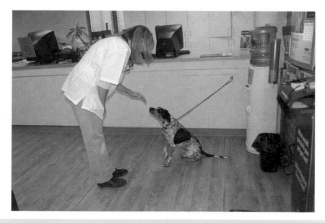

Fig. 8. Walking directly toward the dog and reaching over the dog's head can be threatening to a dog. In this picture, the dog is not retreating but is showing fear to the approach.

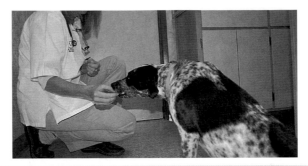

Fig. 9. Kneeling sideways to the dog and offering it treats to encourage it to come to the examiner versus approaching the pet frontally and reaching over it.

Some patients are much less aggressive in the owner's absence. This possibility always can be suggested without arousing suspicion from the owners after other approaches have failed. If the pet is taken from the owner on the first indication that there may be some aggression, and the owner overhears the pet's crying, barking, or growling, the owner generally assumes the pet is being mishandled. If the owner is able to see at first hand how the animal reacts to nonthreatening approaches and handling, and the animal acts poorly, the owner is less likely to jump to incorrect conclusions when the pet is removed.

For minor to moderate cases of anxiety- and fear-induced aggression, owners can be encouraged to bring the pet's favorite toy to the examination. Stalling the examination periodically to engage the animal in play can be a great way to change the pet's emotion from escalating arousal and aggression to relaxation and friendliness (Fig. 11). Having the owner or technician feed the pet throughout the examination can be helpful for mild to moderately anxious patients (Fig. 12). The owner also might consider bringing along the pet's

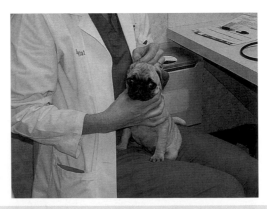

Fig. 10. Small patients can be made more relaxed by setting them on the examiner's lap. The entire physical and vaccinations can be done in this fashion. This method is comforting for both the pet and the owner.

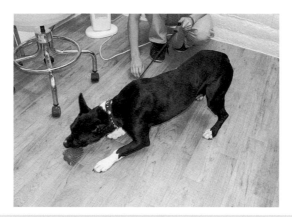

Fig. 11. A dog playing with a toy during an examination.

favorite blanket on which it can lie or in which it might be wrapped during the examination. Some pets might be calmer if some or all of the examination is performed while they remain in their own crates (provided the crate is top opening). The feline cheek gland F3 pheromone (Feliway, Ceva Santé Animale, Libourne, France) or the canine-appeasing pheromone (DAP, Ceva Santé Animale) placed on the pet's blanket or in its crate also may help calm the pet during travel and during the visit [7–9]. A DAP collar may be useful in reducing anxiety beginning with the car trip to the veterinarian [10]. Veterinarians also may consider using DAP or Feliway diffusers in their examination or treatment areas [11].

Occasionally the decision should be made to abandon the examination on that day and to reschedule. The owner may be instructed to give sedatives

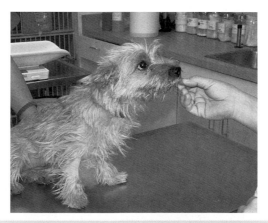

Fig. 12. Feeding the dog or cat during the examination may help alleviate some anxiety and associate the veterinary staff/examination with a positive experience.

or anxiolytic drugs at home before the next appointment or instructed on desensitizing the dog to a basket muzzle. Many modifications to the next visit can be discussed and orchestrated before the animal returns. Consider scheduling that pet at a slower, quieter time of day. Owners can be instructed to have the pet wait in the car while they check in with reception and a room is made available. To avoid the stress and agitation that can develop in a busy waiting room, the pet may be ushered through a side or back door and immediately into an examination room. Occasionally the animal may respond better if met in the parking lot and possibly even examined in this setting. The technician may avoid taking the temperature before the veterinarian examines the animal. One always must remember to document in the pet's chart which techniques were successful. Doing so will save much time and difficulty on the patient's subsequent visits.

If reasonable attempts have been made to work slowly, offer treats, and speak softly to the pet, and the veterinarian or staff still is met with aggression, owners often agree readily to alternative recommendations, including muzzling or other safe restraint tools, separating the pet from the owner during the examination, or using sedatives.

TOOLS

There are many commercially available products for the safer (although not necessarily gentler), handling of aggressive patients, including muzzles (cone, basket, gauze, tape), blankets, bags, nets, leather gloves, Elizabethan collars, rabies poles, pole syringes, snares, squeeze chutes, and induction chambers. Each has advantages and disadvantages, so it is helpful to be familiar with the products, their advantages, and their limitations.

Towels/Blankets

One commonly used and highly effective safety device that may be less confrontational and therefore less fear evoking is a simple blanket or towel placed over and/or around the patient. Blocking visual access often can minimize arousal in many patients, especially cats (Fig. 13). The towel or blanket also serves as a protective barrier between the patient and the handler. A towel can be very effective for muzzle-wise small dogs, often affording the veterinarian enough control to perform a physical examination and blood draw or to administer injectable sedative drugs.

Muzzles

The most common muzzle used for dogs in veterinary practices is the leather or nylon cone-type muzzle that holds the mouth closed. The leather forms are more sturdy and easier to apply when the timing and accuracy of the first placement is crucial (Fig. 14). Other forms include gauze or tape muzzles, which rely on keeping the mouth forcefully closed and inhibit proper panting, which most fearful animals exhibit. Preventing adequate panting further stresses the patient, causing more struggling and sometimes even life-threatening restriction of airflow, especially in the already respiratory-compromised patient. Plastic or

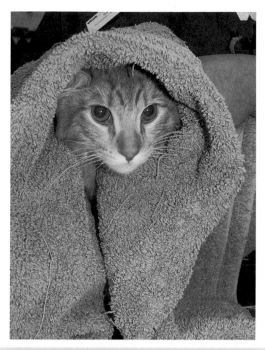

Fig. 13. Restraining a cat in a towel. The towel can be laid over the face to block visual access to help calm the cat and protect the handler.

vinyl-coated wire basket muzzles for dogs are safer and are much preferred to the standard conc-type, gauze, or tape muzzle. The basket configuration allows the animal to pant effectively, which is a safety issue and also may lessen that animal's stress (Fig. 15). The basket muzzle also can be safely left on the pet and the pet then placed in the kennel or cage for later handling. In hot climates or in certain animals, however, the risk of overheating remains, so every animal should be monitored carefully while wearing any muzzle. Every hospital should be equipped with a full set of basket muzzles for in-hospital use and may consider providing them for sale to clients. Owners of clinic-aggressive dogs should be advised how to desensitize their dog to the basket muzzle at home over several weeks and then should apply the muzzle before leaving the home for the next veterinary visit. A ball-type head device (Air Muzzle, SmartPractice, Phoenix, Arizona) also is available for small dogs and cats. This air muzzle can be applied more safely, because the hands are protected behind the device. Once on the pet, it allows the patient full, normal breathing with minimal stress. The blue shield blocks the animal's ventral vision to aid in jugular venipuncture (Fig. 16). Its use is limited to smaller patients. Although it is lightweight, it can be a bit bulky for the smallest of patients. Cat muzzles can be used to cover the mouth and eyes, both for safety and to obscure the visual threat of the stimulus while the neck is accessed for jugular venipuncture.

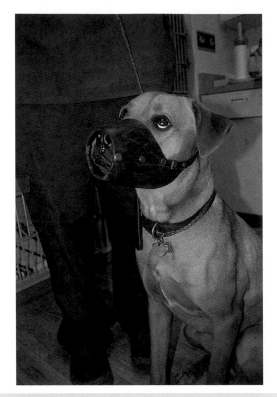

Fig. 14. A leather cone-type muzzle.

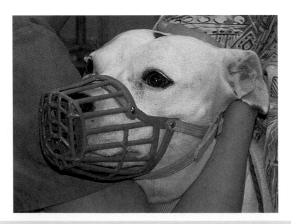

Fig. 15. A vinyl basket muzzle.

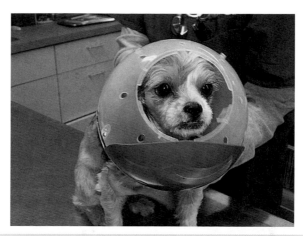

Fig. 16. The Air Muzzle (SmartPractice, Phoenix, Arizona) is helpful in dealing with small dogs and cats (generally less than 12 pounds). It also can be fitted with an oxygen-line adaptor to deliver oxygen or gas anesthesia.

Additional restraint of the remainder of the body might require the use of a blanket or towel also. The use of a muzzle often allows the veterinarian and staff to work more calmly around the pet, which itself may help calm the pet. In addition, if the procedure evokes little or no discomfort, and the pet learns that aggressive displays are no longer successful in removing the stimulus, the pet may become calmer.

Head collars (Gentle Leader, Premier Pet Products, Richmond, Virginia) also can be used in mild to moderately aggressive dogs (Fig. 17). The head

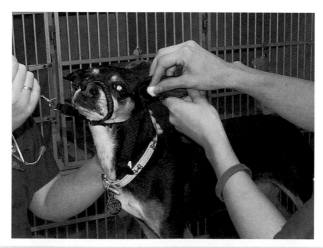

Fig. 17. Using a head collar to restrain a dog for ear cleaning. The head collar is held forward to prevent the dog's head (and mouth) from moving toward the examiner.

collar allows the experienced handler to control the head effectively for a simple examination by the veterinarian. Head collars do not cause any discomfort and often can be more relaxing than other products or handling techniques. This tool works best for dogs that already are used to the head collar and are wearing it to the hospital visit. The head halter also provides an opportunity to reinforce desirable behavior by releasing tension on the mouth and by offering favored food treats if the dog is sufficiently motivated.

Nets

Nets such as the Extendible Capture Net (Campbell Pet Products, Brush Prairie, Washington) or a converted bass fishing net can be very effective for catching extremely aggressive or feral cats safely. Handling the nets effectively requires a little practice, but once the technique is mastered it is easy and effective (Fig. 18). Cats seem to have far less stress in this restraint device than with more forceful physical handling and restraint (which often includes holding the cat by the scruff of the neck). It also is far safer for the handler. The clamshell-type net is effective also, but "catching" the cat is a little more awkward because of the large frame (Fig. 19). Nets do not allow a physical examination but can provide quick and effective restraint to inject sedatives.

Other Tools

An Elizabethan collar or "e-collar" can offer sufficient control to work safely and calmly around some dogs and cats because some procedures then can be performed while protected from the mouth. The e-collar should extend several inches past the muzzle for the best results. Of course, its use is an option only if the e-collar can be fitted successfully and the procedures do not involve treatment or handling of the face or muzzle. The Calming Cap (Premier Pet

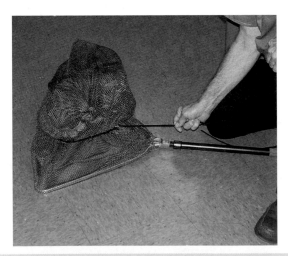

Fig. 18. A net device useful in catching and restraining extremely fearful cats.

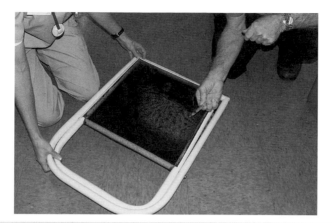

Fig. 19. Clamshell-type net.

Products, Midlothian, Virginia) also may be effective for mild to moderately anxious or agitated pets (Fig. 20). This cap reduces visual stimuli by essentially filtering the dog's vision through a sheer fabric panel. It can be used for nail trims, blood draws, and other situations in which the animal may be excessively visually stimulated.

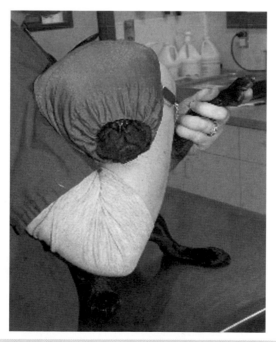

Fig. 20. The Calming Cap from Premier Pet Products (Richmond, Virginia) can be used for some pets to help calm/quiet them for procedures such as nail trims and blood draws.

Less Desirable Options

Leather gloves are still used frequently in the clinic and can be effective in retrieving/holding the smaller patients but are very limiting for the handler. They also seem to be stressful for the patient, so a towel may be a far more appropriate option. (For extra protection, gloves may be used with the towel.) Rabies poles should be used as infrequently as possible. These poles are easily abused by the staff and can be very dangerous if the pole is older and is not working smoothly or is used by an inexperienced handler. These poles are threatening and frightening to the animal and are useful only for protecting the handler against an extremely dangerous dog. In most cases, a more humane and less threatening option can be found.

Induction chambers have been used for both small dogs and cats. The pets can be "poured" into the chamber from their carrier and anesthetic gases hooked up to the box (Fig. 21). Their use is discouraged because of the increased dangers to the patient and increased exposure of the staff to unscavenged anesthetic gases. The animals show significant cardiovascular stress as shown by more profound hypotension and hypoventilation noted at the depth of anesthesia required for intubation, and the isoflurane is an irritant to the mucous membranes (Victoria Lukasic, DVM, Tucson, Arizona, personal communication, 2006). Therefore other forms of chemical restraint are preferred.

CHEMICAL RESTRAINT

Many veterinarians believe it is acceptable to use heavy restraint or punitive measures with problem patients to succeed with a particular examination/procedure. This approach is not advisable for many reasons, including the

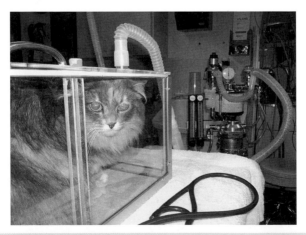

Fig. 21. Induction chambers should be avoided because of the increased risks to the animal and exposure of the staff to unscavenged anesthetic gases.

possibility of injury to the patient, injury to the staff, accelerated aggression on subsequent visits, ethical obligations, and legal liability of abuse. In addition, struggling with an aggressive patient and the subsequent catecholamine release has been reported to cause myocardial necrosis and death of the patient [12]. If gentle handling techniques or some combination of the previously mentioned handling products prove unsuccessful to allow a safe examination/procedure, the use of pharmacologic restraint should be discussed with the owner (Table 1). In fact, except for procedures that are quick and relatively painless, anxiolytics and chemical restraint may be preferable to any type of restraint or product that might cause excessive anxiety or aggression. The following are suggestions of drugs that might be effective. These lists are far from comprehensive and are simply suggestions. Each case needs to be treated individually taking into consideration age, concurrent disease processes, and the pet's previous medical history.

Pharmacologic Restraint
Benzodiazepines
Benzodiazepines are centrally acting muscle relaxants and anxiolytic drugs and can be very effective in minimizing the anxiety of a veterinary visit. They may be given as an injection or orally. Oral benzodiazepines, given before the visit, may be sufficient to reduce anxiety associated with travel and veterinary handling in some pets and may increase the possibility that food counterconditioning might be successful. In addition, benzodiazepines might have an amnesic effect so that the pet does not remember an unpleasant procedure. One concern for this class of drug is a paradoxical response seen in some dogs and cats (excitement, restlessness, insomnia). In addition, although benzodiazepines may reduce fear and anxiety in pets that are displaying aggression, some pets may become more aggressive because of disinhibition if the fear has been inhibiting their aggressive response [13]. For injection, midazolam is recommended over diazepam for its ability to be absorbed after intramuscular administration. Benzodiazepines alone seldom are sufficient in a pet that is highly fearful or aggressive. Injectable benzodiazepines also have the advantage of reversibility with the drug flumazenil.

Pre-visit oral dosing:

> Alprazolam (dog): 0.02–0.1 mg/kg PO 30–60 minutes prior to leaving home
> Diazepam (dog): 0.5–2 mg/kg PO 30–60 minutes prior to leaving home
> For injectable dosing and combinations, see Table 1.

Acepromazine
A phenothiazine neuroleptic agent, acepromazine also can be given orally or by injection. This drug generally is a good choice at low doses in combination with other drugs but can increase sensitivity to noise and may lead to unpredictable behavior if used as a sole agent. Highly agitated animals can overcome its effects, and there are reports of increased aggression with acepromazine alone [13]. Therefore, it is prudent to avoid the use of a phenothiazine alone before

Table 1
Examples of effective drug combinations for the difficult to handle patient

Patient group	Drug combinations	Dose[a,b,c,d]	Notes
Difficult dogs	Butorphanol	0.2 mg/kg	Helpful for short procedures such as nail trims, x-rays, blood draws, etc.
	Medetomidine	0.001–0.010 mg/kg	
	Midazolam	0.05–0.2 mg/kg	
Dogs requiring more sedation	Butorphanol	0.2 mg/kg	These dogs require higher medetomidine doses.
	Medetomidine	0.010–0.020 mg/kg	For painful procedures: consider adding buprenorphine 0.02–0.04 mg/kg or substituting the butorphanol or buprenorphine with either morphine 0.5–1.0 mg/kg or hydromorphone 0.1–0.2 mg/kg
	Midazolam	0.05–0.2 mg/kg	
	Telazol[e]	1–2 mg/kg	
Difficult cats	Butorphanol	0.2 mg/kg	Helpful for short procedures such as nail trims, x-rays, blood draws, etc.
	Medetomidine	0.001–0.015 mg/kg	
	Midazolam	0.05–0.2 mg/kg	
Cats requiring more sedation	Butorphanol	0.2 mg/kg	These cats require higher medetomidine doses.
	Medetomidine	0.015–0.020 mg/kg	Add ketamine only if insufficient sedation from opioid, higher dose medetomidine, and midazolam.
	Midazolam	0.05–0.2 mg/kg	For painful procedures: consider adding buprenorphine 0.02–0.04 mg/kg or substituting the butorphanol or buprenorphine with either morphine at 0.5 mg/kg or hydromorphone at 0.1 mg/kg
	Ketamine	1–5 mg/kg	

All procedural sedation doses are given intramuscularly.

This list is far from comprehensive. Appropriate selection should be made for the individual patient, and one must consider underlying health conditions and age, and the procedures for which the drugs are to be used. Further information can be obtained from http://www.vasg.org.

[a]Dose to lean body weight estimate.

[b]If medications are given prior to patient arrival, adjust above doses based on prior medication effects.

[c]For comparable dexemedtomidine dosing, reduce the above medetomidine doses by half (drug volume remains the same).

[d]Consider the use of 0.1 mg/mL medetomidine and low-dose insulin syringes when dosing small patients.

[e]Add Telazol only if insufficient sedation from opioid, higher dose medetomidine, and midazolam.

Courtesy of the Veterinary Information Network, Davis, CA; with permission.

a veterinary visit, because it does not reduce anxiety and can lead to hypotension and bradycardia that may interfere with the use of more effective injectable drugs. It may reduce nausea associated with car rides, however, and may be sufficient to allow safe and gentle restraint for preventive car visits in healthy pets. Whether alone or as part of a combination therapy, injectable acepromazine likely has little value in cats. Doses of acepromazine (per PromAce package insert, Fort Dodge Animal Health, Fort Dodge Iowa) are:
   Pre-visit oral dosing

> Acepromazine (dog): 0.55–2.2 mg/kg by mouth
> Cat: 1.1–2.2 mg/kg by mouth
> For injectable dosing and combinations, see Table 1.

Combination Oral Therapy

Where additional oral sedation is required prior to the visit, acepromazine and a benzodiazepine may be used concurrently, provided there are no contraindications for either of the products. For other combinations of oral agents, which may be a consideration for the highly aggressive dog, some additional off label suggestions are available at http://www.vasg.org/oral_sedation_for_difficult_dogs.htm. Although the safety of owners, veterinarians, and staff are a primary concern, informed consent is essential when these off label combinations are used.

Injectable Medications

Opioids

Butorphanol, buprenorphine. These are partial opiate agonists mostly used in an injectable form and are safe and effective when used in combination with other drugs such as medetomidine and midazolam. However, butorphanol and buprenorphine are difficult to reverse if undesired effects occur. Butorphanol is suited only to procedural sedation, because it lacks significant analgesic properties. Buprenorphine is well suited to mild to moderate pain but has delayed onset time. In addition, buprenorphine has little to no inherent sedative effects compared to other opioids. For injectable dosing and combinations, see Table 1.

Morphine, hydromorphone. These are full mu agonists, which are also safe and effective when used in combination with other drugs such as medetomidine and midazolam. Mu agonists are an excellent choice for any sedative event and also provide an opportunity for reversal if indicated or if necessary. They are well suited to the management of all pain levels. Patients receiving mu agonists likely will experience transient nausea and may experience unwanted post-sedation dysphoria. For injectable dosing and combinations, see Table 1.

Medetomidine or dexmedetomidine

This is an alpha$_2$ adrenergic agonist injectable that can be used as to aid in restraint for examination and minor procedures. Highly agitated animals may appear refractory to the drug, however, and responses appear to be variable. The drug should not be re-dosed (it is advised that agitated dogs be allowed to rest quietly before administration of the drug). Medetomidine is used best in combination with other agents and should be used only in healthy pets with no evidence of cardiac compromise or other major systemic disease. The ability to reverse the drug with atipamezole is another advantage to using medetomidine. For injectable dosing and combinations, see Table 1.

Ketamine

Ketamine is a dissociative general anesthetic that can be given intramuscularly to aggressive cats if they can be restrained sufficiently in a blanket, fishnet, or clamshell type device. For highly aggressive cats, 1 mL of ketamine can be sprayed into the open mouth or directed into the cat's mouth using a feline urethral catheter through the cage bars. The drug should be sprayed quickly so the cat does not chew and swallow the catheter. Once the cat can be more safely handled, medetomidine IM can be administered for more effective sedation and control. Ketamine is suited most for use in a low dose combination with medetomidine and an opioid. Telazol is a prepared combination of teletamine and zolazepam, and therefore, has similar properties to combining midazolam and ketamine. For injectable dosing and combinations, see Table 1.

Injectable delivery of drugs

Once the decision is made to give injectable sedation to a problem patient, the technique of administration needs to be decided. In the smaller patients, muzzling and physical restraint may be adequate, and a towel or blanket may aid in controlling them. These techniques are not necessarily effective in large dogs, however, and often a muzzle cannot be applied by either the owner or the technical staff. Drugs should be given when the dog or cat is least excitable, perhaps immediately upon entering the clinic, and when there are few if any other distractions in the waiting room. If the dog or cat already is highly aroused and defensive, the drug therapy is unlikely to be fully successful. These patients can be asked to come back on another day, and the staff can be prepared to administer the drugs immediately. If safety is not a factor, or the dog is muzzled, the injection might be given with the owner assisting in restraint while the injection is administered. Occasionally the large dog can be tricked into "leaving" the examination room, and the injection can be administered quickly into the flank or sublumbar muscles while it is walking through the door with its owner or a technician. If this approach is unsuccessful, a door and wall can be used as a squeeze chute, pulling the leash through the gap and holding the dog's head in this position while the door is held against the patient and the injection administered in the lumbar or flank muscles. A pole syringe also can be used, keeping the handler far enough away to avoid serious injury. Similarly, for cats that have been brought into the clinic in a carrier or blanket, it might be easiest to give the injection while the cat is still wrapped or by removing the top of the carrier, rather than stressing the animal by removing it from this protection. If a muzzle has not been applied already, it might be applied as soon as the sedation begins to take effect.

SUMMARY

Although it is frustrating for an appointment to be held up by an aggressive pet, and the staff begins to lose patience with the animal, there is little or no advantage in using excessive force and anger with these pets. If this approach is used, the animal probably will escalate its aggression toward the handlers, and the risk of injuries to the handlers or pet is increased. These patients also are more likely to be more aggressive on subsequent visits, and the owners will believe the staff has abused their pet. To work better with patients it is important to recognize fear in the dogs and cats that visit a clinic and to understand that such fear is the motivating factor for most of the aggression seen in the veterinary clinic. Teaching the staff how to minimize the stimuli and situations that lead to fear will help create a more relaxed and enjoyable atmosphere for all involved. By adopting and practicing a calmer and less forceful way of handling patients, the welfare of the pets will be greatly improved, and the owner will be bonded more strongly to that veterinary team.

References

[1] Blanchard DC, Blanchard RJ. Stress and aggressive behaviors. In: Nelson RJ, editor. Biology of aggression. New York: Oxford University Press; 2006. p. 275.

[2] Overall KL. Fears, anxieties and stereotypes. In: Overall KL, editor. Clinical behavioral medicine for small animals. St. Louis: Mosby; 1997. p. 213.

[3] Yin S. Simple handling techniques for dogs. Compend Contin Educ Vet 2007;29(6):352–8.

[4] Lindsay SR. Aggressive behavior: basic concepts and principles. In: Lindsay SR, editor, Handbook of applied dog behavior and training. vol 2. Ames (IA): Iowa State University Press; 2001. p. 171.

[5] Landsberg GM, Hunthausen W, Ackerman L. Stereotypic and compulsive disorders. In: Landsberg GM, Hunthausen W, Ackerman L, editors. Handbook of behavior problems of the dog and cat. 2nd edition. Edinburgh: W.B Saunders; 2003. p. 198–9.

[6] Lindsay SR. Excessive behavior. In: Lindsay SR, editor, Handbook of applied dog behavior and training. vol 2. Ames (IA): Iowa State University Press; 2001. p. 135.

[7] Cerissa A, Griffith CA, Steigerwald ES, et al. Effects of a synthetic facial pheromone on behavior of cats. J Am Vet Med Assoc 2000;217:1154–6.

[8] Gaultier E, Pageat P, Tessier Y. Effect of a feline appeasing pheromone analogue on manifestations of stress in cats during transport. Proceedings of 32nd International Society for Applied Ethology. Clermont-Ferrand 1998.

[9] Gaultier E, Pageat P. Effects of a synthetic dog appeasing pheromone (DAP) on behaviour problems during transport. In: Seksel K, editor. Proc 4th IVBM. Sydney (Australia): Post Graduate Foundation in Veterinary Science; 2003. p. 33–5.

[10] Estelles MG, Mills DS. Signs of travel-related problems in dogs and their response to treatment with dog-appeasing pheromone. Vet Rec 2006;159:140–8.

[11] Mills DS, Ramos D, Estelles MG, et al. A triple blind placebo-controlled investigation into the assessment of the effect of Dog Appeasing Pheromone (DAP) on anxiety related behaviour of problem dogs in the veterinary clinic. Appl Anim Behav Sci 2006;98:114–26.

[12] Pinson D. Myocardial necrosis and sudden death after an episode of aggressive behavior in a dog. J Am Vet Med Assoc 1997;211:1371–2.

[13] Overall K. Behavioral pharmacology. In: Overall KL, editor. Clinical behavioral medicine for small animals. St. Louis: Mosby; 1997. p. 307.

Vet Clin Small Anim 38 (2008) 1005–1021

VETERINARY CLINICS
SMALL ANIMAL PRACTICE

ELSEVIER
SAUNDERS

Managing Pets with Behavior Problems: Realistic Expectations

Debra F. Horwitz, DVM

Veterinary Behavior Consultations, 11469 Olive Boulevard #254, St. Louis, MO 63141-7108, USA

OVERVIEW

Behavior problems are a source of distress for owners and often for veterinarians when they are first presented with the problem in the examination room. Time constraints, personal interest, or lack of knowledge may preclude a full examination and consultation. Despite these limitations, veterinarians should make every effort to provide guidance about how the owners might prevent the problem from continuing or proceed to improve the problem.

A separate appointment time is the best way to offer management recommendations. This approach allows evaluation of the problem so that the most appropriate recommendations can be made.

WHAT DO MANAGEMENT SOLUTIONS OFFER?

In most cases behavior problems, by the time they are mentioned to the veterinarian, are not isolated events. In fact, they are likely to occur fairly frequently, often causing distress to the owner and pet alike. Behavior problems often are cited as a reason for pet relinquishment [1–5], and it is likely that if the pet is not euthanized it will re-homed and perhaps exhibit the same behavior in the new home [6]. Management solutions can help break the cycle of frustration and, in the case of aggression, perhaps prevent further injuries to people and other animals.

Management solutions also prevent further learning from making the problem worse. Each time the pet engages in the unwanted behavior, that behavior is further reinforced and shaped. Often careful questioning finds that the pet is selecting the behavior increasingly earlier in the behavioral sequence, and the undesirable behavior itself can escalate over time. Behaviors that are repeated may bias neurologic pathways to select that response at the next encounter with the stimulus [7]. The escalation of the problem behavior often coincides with increased owner attempts to stop and/or change the behavior. These interventions can be punitive, dangerous, and damaging to the human–animal bond and may further increase anxiety and conflict. By managing the situation

E-mail address: debhdvm@aol.com

doi:10.1016/j.cvsm.2008.04.006

and decreasing the occurrences of the problem behaviors, a certain sense of order can be restored. (For additional details on conflict and aggression, see the article by Luescher and Reisner in this issue.)

Management solutions also allow the owner to acknowledge and respect the individual pet's limitations. In many cases the pet does not have a problem with its behavior because it has a goal in performing the behavior, whether or not that goal is understandable or acceptable to the owner. The dog that barks and lunges at people or other dogs usually wants them to stay away, and of course they do. Because the behavior is successful, the likelihood that the behavior will be repeated in similar circumstances is increased. If a situation is likely to evoke a certain response, especially one that triggers fear or anxiety, either ending or avoiding that situation should diminish the underlying emotion.

Finally, management interventions may help decrease emotional arousal. When a pet is highly emotionally aroused and displaying aggression, anxiety, fear, or some other emotion, it is unable to learn something new. In fact, teaching the pet new and appropriate tasks is impractical at the time the problem behavior is being exhibited. If the problem behavior is going to change, however, new tasks must be taught so that the pet learns to perform an alternative behavior that is acceptable to the owner when presented with the stimulus in the future. Therefore, having strategies to avoid and/or remove the pet from the situation can help keep emotional arousal low, might provide an opportunity to train behaviors that are desirable, and perhaps might diminish future episodes, increasing safety and reducing anxiety for the owner and pet.

GETTING STARTED

At each veterinary visit owners should be questioned about whether the pet has exhibited any changes in behavior or any behavioral issues that they might want to address. Pet owners otherwise may not be aware that the veterinarian is available and willing to provide guidance or may wait until the problem is well established and potentially more difficult to manage or treat (see the article by Shaw and colleagues elsewhere in this issue). Once a client has mentioned a behavioral issue, the first step is to acknowledge quickly that a problem exists and to recognize that intervention is appropriate. A complete physical examination and other laboratory testing or imaging studies as indicated by findings are essential, because illness often can contribute to behavioral problems. Time is necessary to provide the appropriate recommendations and interventions; therefore separate appointments should be scheduled. The veterinarian should make clear to the client the goal for the appointment. If full behavioral consultations are offered, set aside enough time to do so. The articles by Seibert and Landsberg and Shaw and colleagues found elsewhere in this issue detail how that might be accomplished. If a full consultation is beyond the veterinarian's expertise, one should offer an appointment that will focus on help managing the problem behavior and allow at least an hour. Before beginning, explain charges to the client and how follow-up will be obtained. Plan to make a chart or history form so that the consultation and resultant recommendations are recorded.

Handouts, training aids, books, and videos are all useful adjuncts to creating a management plan. Having these tools ready in the consultation location will allow efficient use of the clinician's time. Head collars, body harnesses, muzzles, pheromones, and even certain toys can be stocked and ready to be dispensed. Handouts and books are available from many sources, and a well-stocked library is useful. Providing useful Web links also can help support or even expand the veterinarian's recommendations after the visit.

In some cases the situation has entered a crisis mode, and clients cannot wait for an appointment. One of the more useful interventions for many behaviors is to offer to get the animal out of the home, either with day boarding or 24-hour care. If the problem is aggression, and injuries have occurred, removing the animal from the home may allow decisions to be made and provide safety for people who would have come in contact with the dog. If the problem is separation anxiety with destruction to property and/or injury to the animal, day boarding allows all parties to become calm and perhaps reach some sort of equilibrium. If the clinic is unable to offer these options, one should become familiar with trustworthy kennels in the area to which clients can be referred for these interventions.

DIAGNOSIS

At the appointment it is essential to identify the problem behavior(s) that need to be addressed. As straightforward as this process may seem, in many cases the client's description of the problem may be filled with emotional statements and have very little description of actual behaviors. For example, a client may come with the complaint of an overreaction to noises such as the telephone ringing or the doorbell. When asked what the animal does, the owner replies that when the telephone rings and the owner gets up to answer it, the dog chases and nips at them. If, however, they answer the telephone sitting down or are next to the telephone when it rings, the problem does not occur. In this case the problem is not the ringing of the telephone but rather the movement that answering the telephone or moving toward the door elicits. Therefore, an accurate description helps determine what types of intervention might be useful. In this example, keeping the telephone nearby (eg, by carrying a portable phone) might be one management tool.

In addition it is necessary to attempt to establish the frequency of the problem behavior so that progress can be assessed. Improvement is more difficult to track in problems that occur with low frequency, because a lack of problematic behavior may not mean the target behavior has changed, but rather that it has not yet occurred. If possible, knowing when and where the behavior takes place can point to management techniques that might be effective interventions.

The next step is to attempt to identify inciting stimuli whenever possible. Owner descriptions may link together various things that may not be related. Destruction in the absence of the owner is a good example. The owners may relate that when they leave the home the dog gets into the garbage and/or the pantry and creates a mess. This behavior could appear to be separation anxiety, but careful questioning might reveal that the dog does the same thing when they are home if they do not watch the pet. In this case the problem might be food-seeking behavior, and making a video or audiotape might be needed to determine what is happening and if any signs of anxiety are noted. If none are seen, then putting food and garbage in inaccessible locations may manage the behavior.

Owner descriptions often are peppered with emotional phrases such as "he looks upset," "he is afraid," "he looks angry," or "he is mad at me." These statements are not helpful unless they can be coupled with descriptions of actions and body postures. Descriptions of actions and postures allow the clinician to attempt to assess the underlying emotional state of the pet, which may or may not correspond to the owners' statements. This assessment becomes essential, especially in behavioral problems with underlying anxiety, because treatment must focus on changing the emotional state as well as the pet's outward behavior. The goal of the interview is to learn what the animal did, what it looked like both at the present time and at the time the behavior first began, and not what the owner thought the pet "meant" by its behavior.

Understanding the personality/temperament of the pet also is important when working on management solutions and managing expectations. Highly excitable and reactive pets may find certain stimuli always difficult to cope with. Some animals may do better by always being confined when large numbers of people come to the home or by not going to the dog park. Helping owners understand the individual pet's limitations can help set realistic expectations for success.

PROGNOSIS

For rehabilitation of the pet to be successful, most behavior problems require a time commitment from the family and willingness to alter the daily routine. In some cases the family composition, the time available, and frustration with the ongoing problem may impede resolution. In certain cases the owners may be more willing to work for change if management solutions can diminish the problem behavior. Behaviors that have been present for some time may be more difficult to eliminate, so prognosis might be improved by focusing on improvement rather than resolution.

ASSESSING PROGNOSIS FOR AGGRESSIVE DOGS

The commonly used factors in assessing risk and prognosis for aggression in dogs include the willingness of the owners to live with risk, the family composition, the ability to provide safety, the size of the pet, the predictability of the behavior, the context, the choices the pet made, and, in cases of aggression, the severity of the aggression and the injuries sustained.

Depending on the circumstances, their temperament, genetic factors, and experiences, all pets can bite. When an animal chooses to use aggression in a certain situation, then, at least in that situation, aggressive biting is a behavioral strategy that individual pet is willing to use. If successful, aggression is likely to be repeated, should that situation recur in the future. For this reason an animal that has bitten in the past usually presents a higher risk for future biting than one that never has bitten anyone. Owners need to realize that the risk of future biting is real, and some owners may not be willing to live with that risk. Biting animals are rarely cured; rather, they are controlled and with proper safety precautions may be able to be retained in the home.

Certain family compositions may make keeping an aggressive pet unsafe. Families with very small children, elderly persons, and persons who have physical or mental disabilities or a very unpredictable household schedule may not be suitable for rehabilitating an aggressive pet. Because the possibility of future biting events is real, some households may not be able to provide safety for people who live there or come to visit the home.

The size of the pet also is a factor in assessing prognosis in aggression cases because larger dogs tend to do more damage when and if they bite. In a study looking at risk factors for euthanasia in dogs that were aggressive toward family members, a dog weighing more than 18 kg was more likely to be euthanized than a smaller dog, especially if the aggression was shown in what were considered "benign dominance challenges such as petting and bending over the dog" [8]. Later research looking at the risk factors for dog bites to owners in a household setting, however, found that small dogs were more likely than larger dogs to have bitten family members [9]. Some homes may tolerate aggressive behaviors from smaller dogs because of a perception that they may not be as dangerous.

Another factor that must be considered when determining risk and prognosis is the predictability of when and how aggressive the pet might be in response to certain triggers. Reisner and colleagues [8] found that dogs whose aggressive behaviors were unpredictable more likely to be euthanized than dogs who were predictable. In other words, if the dog growls only when one tries to move it, the situation might be sufficiently predictable and preventable that it might be possible to keep the dog in the home. On the other hand, a dog that sometimes growls and at other times lunges and bites when presented with the same trigger stimulus might have to be relinquished. Predictability may make it easier for some owners to avoid the aggressive encounters and to diminish biting behavior and subsequent injury.

The context in which the aggression occurs is another factor to consider. In some contexts aggression is understandable, although unwanted. These contexts include handling food, painful manipulations, extremely frightening situations, and redirected aggression. In some cases it may be possible to manage these situations, diminish pain, or avoid the situation and/or medicate the animal.

It also helps to look at the choices that the dog has made during these episodes and at the severity of the aggressive behavior that occurred. Many dogs have good control of their aggressive signaling and can choose various levels with which to respond. Aggressive responses can vary from threats (growling, snarling with or without a growl), snapping (bites that do not make contact), bites without puncture or laceration, and injurious, damaging bites. Historical information gathered during a behavioral consultation should attempt to determine if the dog had other choices during the encounter (such as escape, lower-level aggressive response), whether the dog signaled to show intent before aggression, whether the response was out of proportion to the supposed stimulus, and if the aggressive behavior has changed over time. Finally, the severity of the injuries inflicted should be evaluated. In some situations the dog may give only a single bite; other dogs may bite multiple times within a single episode. In some situations the biting might be directed toward the stimulus (a hand reaching for the dog); in other cases the pet may attack other body parts (jumping up at the torso or face). More extreme responses and severe injuries requiring medical attention may be associated with greater risk and poorer prognosis. Pets that show very explosive aggressive responses, especially in response to low-level stimuli, may be particularly dangerous to keep in the home.

AGGRESSION AND SAFETY

Because aggressive behavior is a common owner complaint, and the risk of human or animal injury might be high, instructions for providing safety for those who must be around the pet are essential and should be the first issue addressed. Owners should be informed that all animals may bite at some time, and that those that are known to have used biting as a strategy in the past may be more likely to do so in the future. Often the only way to prevent all future aggressive episodes and injury is euthanasia especially if re-homing is impractical or unsafe.

Education on how pets display aggressive signaling using facial expressions and body postures should be explained and described to owners. A better understanding of what aggressive signaling looks like and what the animal is trying to convey often helps owners avoid injuries. Owners should be advised to discontinue all interactions with animals showing aggressive posturing and not to resume interactions until the animal is calm. Isolation of the pet in a secure location for quite some time may be necessary. Pictures of body postures used by dogs and cats are useful in helping owners understand what they are seeing. These pictures are available from various sources [10,11] and in the article by Levine elsewhere in this issue.

All known trigger situations for aggression must be avoided. A good history should elucidate what these situations and triggers are. If needed, a list should be compiled to clarify for the owner which situations are potentially dangerous. Environmental management, such as separation of individuals from the pet, confinement, and the use of muzzles, leashes and head collars, all factor into providing safety for people around an aggressive pet. In many cases providing safety may mean confining the pet away from either the triggers and/or the victims. The pet should be confined by an adult to a location such as a crate, a room with a lock, or a locked yard from which the dog cannot escape. Confinement must occur each and every time the trigger for the aggression might be encountered; however, many families are unable to take this measure. In addition, all physical reprimands must be stopped, because they are likely to increase the dog's emotional arousal and perhaps its aggressive responses. Specific recommendations for certain situations are described later.

SETTING REALISTIC EXPECTATIONS FOR IMPROVEMENT

Understandably, owners are quite concerned about whether the unwanted behaviors can be curtailed and resolved. Setting realistic expectations for improvement and discussing the difference between improvement and resolution is important. Most behavior problems presented for help may be chronic in nature and in this way may mimic many other chronic disorders seen in veterinary medicine. Often the animals are responding to the social and physical environment in which they live, following their innate tendencies for responses and acclimation. Learning and adaptation also often are responsible for the ongoing performance of the target behavior. Owners should be counseled that behavior problems will take time to control and/or resolve; even after treatment certain problem situations or actions may remain but, it is hoped, will be manifest at a lower level or be easier to control. Asking owners to keep journals and/or daily diaries to assess the frequency of the targeted problem behaviors can help determine if improvement has occurred.

MANAGEMENT OPTIONS

Certain management options may apply to all cases; others are appropriate only in certain situations. In all cases, increasing the owner's understanding of the pet's behavior and of how learning influences later behavior will help the owner view the situation in a more positive way. Some management options require pretraining to increase compliance, as described later. Teaching new responses is the ultimate goal of behavior therapy and usually is facilitated by the use of rewards. It should be determined which rewards are the most desirable for the pet. For most pets, the most desired reward is a food item, but some might prefer play or petting. These rewards should be arranged in a hierarchy, with the most desirable reward reserved for each new task in training that gradually approximates the final goal. No rewards of any kind should be given randomly; rewards must be earned by completion of a requested task.

As part of management, the owner should be educated on ways to provide appropriate and species-specific environmental enrichment and daily exercise. For dogs these might be walks off the property if the pet is under control and play time such as fetch using two objects. For cats, opportunities to forage for food, increased play and hiding, climbing, and jumping opportunities should be provided. All these enrichments can help relieve underlying anxiety and stress that contribute to behavior problems. During interactive times, these activities also can be part of training opportunities and teach the pet appropriate interactions with family members.

Certain management options can be detrimental to the pet or impede resolution; these must be identified and stopped. Repeated encounters with provocative stimuli in an attempt to "socialize" the pet actually may make the pet more sensitive to the stimulus and worsen rather than improve the situation. Therefore, these encounters must be curtailed. Examples include ongoing visits to the dog park with a dog that shows anxious or aggressive responses, allowing people to greet anxious and/or aggressive dogs, or keeping aggressive dogs in a home together despite fighting.

Punishment, especially for aggressive signaling, can be dangerous. The punishment is directed toward the outward signal that the pet is performing, in many cases the aggressive signal. Although the aggressive signal may cease, the underlying emotional state may remain. The result often is what seems to be unpredictable biting behavior, because the pet's emotional state may be the same or worse, even though it has learned not to growl. In reality, it probably is desirable for aggressive dogs to signal so that people and other animals nearby are aware of the danger that this animal presents and, it is hoped, remain far enough away to avoid injury. (See the American Veterinary Society of Animal Behavior punishment guidelines at www.avsabonline.org.)

Recently, treatment modalities seem to have refocused on procedures that have been designed to gain control of the dog through a dominance paradigm and/or exercises. In most cases these methods do not take into consideration any other underlying emotion, such as fear or anxiety, which are the most common reasons for unwanted behaviors. Instead these techniques often rely on punishment, leash corrections, and yelling, which can increase fear and anxiety and even cause aggression directed toward the person administering the technique. For these reasons such interventions are not recommended and in many cases may be harmful.

Finally, vocal or postural interactions in an attempt to soothe the pet also may be counterproductive. Because soft vocal intonations and petting may resemble praise, it is possible for the pet to assume that it is being rewarded for the behavior it is engaging in at the time. Rather than scolding, coddling, or patting the pet, the owner should try to give the pet a direction with a command such as "sit" or "watch," which, if successful can be reinforced.

Increasing Owner Control

Increasing the owner's control over the pet in daily interactions will help the pet learn to follow owner commands and often empowers owners as they learn to control the pet in benign ways. This technique has been called many things over the years (eg, "nothing in life is free" [12], "learn to earn" [13], "structuring your relationship with your pet" [14], "protocol for deference" [15]), but they all have in common asking a pet to perform an obedience task such as "sit" before the pet receives anything that it wants. In general this approach accomplishes three things. If the pet has been asked to sit (and complies) multiple times in a day, it may learn to comply with the sit command at other times and in other situations. Having the dog in a sitting position increases control. For some pets, learning to obey the command also allows them to learn to take contextual cues from the owner (ie, what should I do now?). Finally, it allows controlled and predictable interactions that may help decrease uncertainty and anxiety. In turn, the dog also gains control and predictability by learning what behaviors earn rewards. Both dogs and cats can be asked to follow this protocol. If the animal does not know the command for "sit," that command can be taught, or another command, such as "wait," can be substituted.

Changing Underlying Emotional State: Teaching Relaxation on Command

Because the goal in the treatment of most problem behaviors is to change the pet's underlying emotional state and response when presented with the stimulus from anxiety and fear to calmness and relaxation, teaching relaxation on command is useful. This technique is not an exercise in "sit" and "stay" but rather is an attempt to get physiologic and postural relaxation under voice command. If that control can be accomplished, the pet can be cued to relax when faced with stimuli that cause emotional arousal. Unless the pet knows how to perform the task without distractions and when calm, it is unlikely that the owner could get the pet to relax when emotionally aroused. To be effective, the owners should be given step-by-step instructions in how to teach and assess relaxation in the pet. Various protocols have been detailed in other sources and called various things [14,15]; all have the goal of teaching the pet how to be calm.

It also can be useful for the owner to use a bed, mat, or rug as the training site. This approach allows the behavior not to be associated only with a specific location; because the object is movable, it can be taken to various rooms and the exercise repeated there as well. The pet should be brought calmly to the training location and asked to "sit" or "down" (depending on what the pet knows and the amount of control needed). A leash, head collar, or body harness may be appropriate in some cases. The pet then is cued to stay and relax. The owner should use the same key words each time. The owner should watch the pet for signs of emotional change toward relaxation. These signs might include relaxing of the eyes or ears, no wagging or twitching tail, putting the head down, and slower respirations, but initially the owner should watch for one change and, when that change is observed, reward the pet with food and praise. The pet then is cued to get up, move, and come back to the settle position again. Training sessions should be quite short, only 5 to 10 minutes. Each session can add progressive signs of relaxation. For some pets massage also can be added as an aid to relaxation. A favored toy or chew or feeding toy might also be used to reinforce use of the area, provided the problem is not one of possessive aggression. For some pets using a crate may be more appropriate for relaxation training.

Avoiding Problem Situations: Teaching Confinement

One of the more useful management options for both dogs and cats is confinement to prevent encounters with the stimulus. It is unrealistic, however, to expect a pet to accept confinement without some type of pretraining. Therefore, a program that teaches the pet how to be confined in a crate, in a room with a closed door, or behind a baby gate will help owners be compliant with this recommendation.

Confinement training should start with the pet and the owner in the same room. If a crate is to be used, and the animal already is comfortable using the crate, the pet should be placed in the crate with a delectable food reward and the door latched. The owner should sit nearby occupied with a quiet task and ignore the pet. After a few minutes, and if the pet is calm and quiet, the pet is released. If a crate is not an option, the same protocol can be practiced with a closed door or a baby gate in the doorway. Gradually the amount of time the pet spends in the location is increased, alternating shorter and longer periods. Time should be increased only if the pet is able to remain calm. Once the pet can be calm with the owner present, short sessions with the owner out of the room can be attempted. The time again must return to very short sessions so that the pet is successful and not anxious. Once the pet learns how to be left alone in confinement when there are no distractions, it is more likely to remain there when placed into confinement at other times. Food rewards or whatever is most desirable to the pet always should be used so the animal continues to associate confinement with a pleasant circumstance. A favored toy, chew bone, or food can be used to reinforce the use of the area as well as to help keep the pet in the location. Finally, the pet can be taught to go to the location with a verbal cue, a hand signal, and a food reward.

Avoiding Triggers for Unwanted Behaviors

Avoiding triggers is another useful management tool. Once the trigger stimuli and how they are encountered have been identified correctly, it may be possible to offer strategies for avoidance. Although it might be practical to improve some of these forms of aggression over time, using reward-based training and proper management devices, the initial focus (and sometimes the permanent focus) should be aimed at avoidance. In other situations, avoidance will prevent reinforcement of the behavior through repetition while new behaviors are substituted.

Food-related aggressive episodes

Most food-related aggressive episodes involve dogs, although at times a cat may guard an object. If the dog stands stiffly, growls, snarls (lifts its lip and shows its teeth), lunges, snaps, or bites when approached while eating or when in possession of a toy, chew bone, or stolen item, this situation must be avoided. If the dog is aggressive around human food, it should not be in the room while food is being prepared and consumed. Children must not walk around the home eating food if the dog is in the house. If the dog is aggressive around its food, then the food is prepared while the dog is outside, is placed in a room with a door that can be locked, and the dog is put into this room. The door is closed and locked, if necessary with a latch up high that cannot be reached by children. The dog is not allowed out until the food is consumed. Once the food is consumed, the dog is allowed out but is put outside or in another room, and then the food bowl can be picked up and put away.

If a dog steals some type of human food, the dog should be allowed to consume the food, and no one should attempt to take it away. To prevent further food-stealing episodes, food must be stored out of the dog's reach, or the dog must be kept out of food-related areas. In some homes having a garbage container under the sink for food garbage only and another for paper and nonfood trash helps prevent food stealing from taking place. If the dog or cat is aggressive over certain items, access to these items must be avoided or allowed only when the animal is securely confined. All food items that are given to the pet must be ones that can be consumed quickly, or the pet must be confined while eating them.

Aggressive responses to family members
If the pet gets stiff, growls, snarls (lifts its lip and shows its teeth), lunges, snaps, or bites during any form of social or physical interaction, these interactions must be identified and avoided by family members and visitors. Possible stimuli include petting, hugging, picking up the dog, grooming, pushing, stepping over it, grabbing it by the collar, wiping its feet, and cleaning its ears, among others. Feet can be cleaned by allowing the dog to remain in a room covered with towels until dry. If the dog must be moved frequently from one place to another, it can drag a leash to facilitate moving the pet without physical contact.

If the pet growls, snarls, lunges, snaps, or bites at children in the home, the pet never should be left alone with the children. All interactions must be supervised by an adult, or the pet must be confined away from children. Even during supervised interactions, all potential triggers must be identified so that they can be prevented or avoided. Alternately, muzzles may be appropriate for dogs in some situations. See the article by Luescher and Reisner elsewhere in this issue for more information on this problem in dogs and the article by Curtis found elsewhere in this issue for problems of feline aggression.

Suggestions for Safe Retrieval of Stolen Items
Many pets, primarily dogs, steal items in the household. Often this behavior results in the owner chasing the pet and eventually cornering the animal. Depending on the outcome of previous encounters (especially if they ended with punishment), the pet may respond aggressively when the person attempts to retrieve the item. Many owners insist on "winning" this encounter despite the animal's signalling that it is willing to bite. A way to retrieve items safely is discussed in the following paragraph.

This method is to be used only by an adult who has control of the dog and should not be used by children in the home. The only reason to attempt to retrieve an item is when an item is potentially dangerous to the dog or is highly valuable to the family. Initially the family member should get a highly valued reward (ie, table food). The pet then is shown the food from 5 to 6 feet away, and the owner gives the command to "come" while showing the pet the food. If the dog leaves the item to approach, the owner should back up, call the dog again, and add, "sit." This process is repeated two or three times without giving the dog the food reward until the dog is at least 15 to 20 feet from the object, preferably in another room. The dog then is given the food reward and, if possible, is taken gently by the collar and put into another room with a closed door or outside. Another option is to target train the dog so that it can be lured with the target instead of the food rewards. The target provides a more immediate pretrained method of teaching the dog to come for food without having to "decide" whether the food is sufficiently valuable. If the dog will not allow touching of the collar, it should not be attempted; rather, one should use another food reward to lead the dog into another room where the pet can be confined. After the dog is securely confined in an area away from the item, the item can be retrieved. Most importantly, the food-for-item exchange must never take place directly in front of the pet, because in most cases the animal will eat the food, return to the item, and perhaps bite the owner as well. This technique should be used only when it is absolutely essential that the item be removed from the pet and will not be effective unless the item offered is more valued than the one the pet has stolen.

Box 1 summarizes the techniques for managing aggression towards familiar people.

Aggressive Responses at Windows, Doors, Fences, and on the Arrival of Unfamiliar People

If territorial responses are problematic and/or extreme, the pet must be kept away from windows, doors, and fences (Box 2). Management might require blocking windows, restricting access to certain parts of the home, going outside with the dog, and/or using a leash and head collar both indoors and outdoors for additional control. The pet must never be left outside when no one is home. The pet (dog or cat) always must be confined before the door is opened.

Box 1: Managing aggression towards familiar people

- Avoid delectable food items except as a means of training and counterconditioning to improve the underlying problem.
- Feed the pet in secure confinement.
- Do not try to take an object from the pet.
- When not confined, the pet should be supervised to prevent stealing. Leaving a leash and head halter on the pet can provide safer and more effective control.
- When it is absolutely necessary to retrieve a stolen item, try to lure the pet at least 6 feet from the item using a food reward or target and then, if possible, confine the pet and go get the item.
- Avoid interactions that cause aggressive responses, including, but not limited to, wiping feet, trimming nails, hugging, pushing, and touching the pet while it is resting.

Box 2: Managing territorial responses at windows, doors, and fences and toward visitors

- Block access to areas where the stimuli are encountered. Cover windows and keep the pet out of rooms with a view to the outdoors.
- Always confine the pet before opening the door. Keep a leash handy nearby to facilitate compliance.
- Do not allow the animal outdoors unattended.
- Use a leash and head halter for additional control. The animal should be handled by an adult.
- Do not use retractable leashes.

Confinement is accomplished most easily by teaching a command that signals the pet to go to the confinement area. This task is practiced when no one is at the door so the pet can follow and obey the command reliably and accept confinement when there is no excitement or visitor. This acceptance increases the likelihood that compliance will occur at other times. If the pet will not go readily but can be led on a leash, a leash should be kept near the door, either draped over a doorknob or on a nearby piece of furniture. See the article by Curtis elsewhere in this issue for information on feline aggression toward strangers.

Aggressive Responses on Walks and Away from Home

Dogs that show aggression toward people or other dogs on walks should not go on walks. If walks cannot be avoided, they should be scheduled at low-traffic times or in areas where people arc less likely to be encountered such as industrial parks (Box 3). Busy neighborhoods, downtown areas, parks, and sporting events must be avoided. If the stimulus is encountered during a walk, no matter how far it is from the owner and pet, they must leave the area quickly but

Box 3: Managing unwanted responses on walks

- Do not use retractable leashes.
- Use head halters or no-pull harnesses.
- Walk only one dog at a time.
- Walk during low-traffic times or in low-traffic areas.
- If the stimulus is encountered, the owner should move the dog out of the situation as soon as it is noted by immediately turning the other way, crossing the street, walking the dog past the stimulus if this can be accomplished with a leash and head halter at sufficient distance to avoid any confrontations, or have the pet sit and focus on the owner (again with a leash and head halter) at a sufficient distance so that the other pet can walk by.
- Avoid yelling, scolding, and leash corrections, which will increase arousal.

calmly by turning around, crossing the street, or entering a yard. See the article by Haug found elsewhere in this issue for more information on treatment.

Fighting Between Companion Dogs Within the Home

When dogs within a household fight, severe injury to one or both dogs and to the humans who attempt to separate them is possible. If two dogs are fighting, the owners should not attempt to separate them by grabbing their collars or necks but rather by picking the dogs up by their back legs and elevating the dog while walking backward. Once the dogs have ceased fighting, they should be separated and kept apart until calm. When the dogs are next introduced, both should be on leashes and under owner control. Head halters and muzzles provide an additional level of safety. The owners should request that the dogs sit or down quietly and see if the animals can be together without showing any aggressive or fearful responses.

Because fights between dogs often are elicited by food, owner attention, and high-arousal situations, these stimuli must be avoided [16]. Each dog should be fed in its own bowl in a separate location, and all food bowls should be picked up and put away once feeding time is over. The owners should attempt to control all interactions with the pets using commands to get the dogs to sit before any activity including petting.

Box 4 summarizes techniques for avoiding fighting between dogs.

Fighting Between Household Cats

When cats fight, they can become quite emotionally aroused, and fighting may continue unless the cats are separated until they calm down. Calming can take several hours to days depending on the temperament of the individual cat. Each cat should have food, water, and a litter box in the confinement area. Introductions through a closed door are a good place to start to assess if the cats are calm enough to see one another. Premature introductions often lead to resumption of fighting, so owners should be advised to keep the cats separated until they are calm and to use food rewards to facilitate re-introduction. See the article by Levine in this issue for more information on anxiety and fear in cats.

Box 4: Management of fighting between dogs

- Dogs should be separated when not supervised.
- Dogs must be separated for feeding and food preparation.
- Avoid high-arousal situations: greetings, going through doorways, answering the door.
- Use only quickly consumable treats, not long-lasting food rewards such as bones.
- Use leashes and tie downs when home to increase control and perhaps diminish fighting.

Problem Litter Box Behavior and Urine Spraying

Litter box problems and urine-spraying problems often respond in some degree to improved litter box hygiene and to increasing the number and placement of litter boxes [17].

For urine spraying, avoiding encounters with outdoor cats by blocking windows or keeping them away from the home is a useful management strategy. In some cases litter box usage problems seem to be associated with agonistic social interactions between cats, so treating those issues, adequate provisioning of resources, and separation of cats may be useful strategies. Preventing access to soiled areas by keeping doors closed and by cleaning soiled areas adequately also may help diminish house soiling.

Box 5 summarizes the management of litter box problems and urine spraying.

Canine House Soiling and Marking

Four important management issues can help improve house soiling and marking in dogs. First, owners must accompany their dogs outdoors to verify outdoor elimination. Unless they go outside with the dog, they have no way of knowing if the dog used the outdoor opportunity to empty its bladder and/or bowel. Second, they must supervise the dog when they are home and the dog is indoors. This supervision may require keeping the dog with them on a leash to avoid wandering and subsequent soiling. If they cannot observe the dog, it should be confined in an area that is easily cleaned. Finally, the owners must search the house daily to determine when and where soiling occurs.

Separation Anxiety and Noise Sensitivities

For some animals that have separation anxiety, offering day boarding until treatment options and/or medication have begun to change behavior is a good solution. For dogs that have noise sensitivities, getting the animal to a darkened area and using some white noise to cover the problematic signs can be useful (Box 6). More details are provided in the article by Simpson and Mills found elsewhere in this issue.

Box 5: Managing litter box problems and urine spraying

- Improve litter box hygiene by daily removal of waste material and weekly cleaning and refilling of boxes.
- Provide an adequate number of boxes at different locations.
- Separate cats that show agonistic interactions.
- Clean soiled areas adequately.
- Block access to soiled areas.

Box 6: Managing reactivity to noises
- Remain calm.
- Avoid punishment or assurance.
- Place pet in a darkened quiet area with an adult.
- Use some type of white noise (fan, loud rock and roll music) to block the sound.

Compulsive Disorders of the Skin and Locomotor Disorders

Research has indicated that compulsive disorders in dogs and cats that are presented as licking or chewing problems must have detailed and perhaps prolonged work-up and treatment before being labeled as compulsive disorders [18–20]. Therefore management entails appropriate medical care. Locomotor disorders may respond to increased control through head collars and a command–response relationship and increased activity and exercise as management options.

CONTROL DEVICES TO ENHANCE MANAGEMENT

Control devices can enhance compliance. These devices include fixed (not retractable) leashes, head halters, body harnesses, crates, and basket muzzles. These items can be used both in the home and outdoors. Care should be exercised when using basket muzzles because of the possibility of overheating, because panting is inhibited to some degree. Pretraining to wear a basket muzzle will aid in compliance and acceptance by both the owner and the pet. Motion sensors with or without a citronella collar can help keep pets out of certain areas (see the articles by Moffat and Haug found elsewhere in this issue for more information on management devices).

The clinician or a staff member should know how to fit these items and how to train dogs to accept them willingly. Many sources exist for the products and for advice on how to fit and use them. Video sources are also available at ABRIonline.org.

SUMMARY

Veterinarians can help clients who have problem pets at many levels. Education allows owners to better understand normal behavior, problem behavior, and the individual pet. Management solutions offer a useful tool for owners faced with behavior issues in their pets and allow veterinarians to intervene at a basic, helpful level. In some cases management steps and control devices improve the behavior and allow increased owner control and a reduction in the problem behavior. In other situations it may be only the first step in a treatment protocol. By offering management solutions, veterinarians can help owners who have problem pets begin on the road to recovery.

References

[1] Salman MD, Hutchinson J, Ruch-Gallie R, et al. Behavioral reasons for relinquishment of dogs and cats to 12 shelters. J Appl Anim Welf Sci 2000;3(2):93–106.

[2] Patronek GJ, Glickman LT, Beck AM, et al. Risk factors for relinquishment of dogs to an animal shelter. J Am Vet Med Assoc 1996;209(3):572–81.

[3] Patronek GJ, Glickman LT, Beck AM, et al. Risk factors for relinquishment of cats to an animal shelter. J Am Vet Med Assoc 1996;209(3):582–8.

[4] Miller DD, Staats SR, Partlo C, et al. Factors associated with the decision to surrender a pet to an animal shelter. J Am Vet Med Assoc 1996;209(4):738–42.

[5] Houpt KA, Honig SU, Reisner IR. Breaking the human-companion animal bond. J Am Vet Med Assoc 1996;208(10):1653–8.

[6] Wells DL, Hepper PG. Prevalence of behaviour problems reported by owners of dogs purchased from an animal rescue shelter. Appl Anim Behav Sci 2000;69:55–65.

[7] Lindsay SR. Neurobiology of behavior and learning. In: Lindsay SR, editor. Applied dog behavior and training. Ames (IA): Iowa State University Press; 2000. p. 73–126.

[8] Reisner IR, Erb HN, Houpt KA. Risk factors for behavior-related euthanasia among dominant aggressive dogs: 110 cases (1989–1992). J Am Vet Med Assoc 1994;205(6):855–63.

[9] Guy NC, Luescher UA, Dohoo SE, et al. Risk factors for dog bites to owners in a general veterinary caseload. Appl Anim Behav Sci 2001;74:29–42.

[10] Shepherd K. Development of behaviour, social behaviour and communication in dogs. In: Horwitz D, Mills D, Heath S, editors. BSAVA manual of canine and feline behavioural medicine. Quedgeley, Gloucester (UK): British Small Animal Veterinary Association; 2002. p. 8–20.

[11] Crowell-Davis SL. Social behaviour, communication and development of behaviour in the cat. In: Horwitz D, Mills D, Heath S, editors. BSAVA manual of canine and feline behavioural medicine. Quedgeley, Gloucester (UK): British Small Animal Veterinary Association; 2002. p. 21–9.

[12] Voith VL, Borchelt PL. Diagnosis and treatment of dominance aggression in dogs. Vet Clin North Am Small Anim Pract 1982;12(4):655–63.

[13] Campbell WE. Behavior problems in dogs. 3rd revised edition. Grants Pass (OR): BehaviorRX Systems; 1999. p. 203.

[14] Horwitz DF, Neilson JC. Appendix D handouts. In: Horwitz DF, Neilson JC, editors. Blackwell's five-minute veterinary consult clinical companion. Ames (IA): Blackwell Publishing; 2007. p. 548–79.

[15] Horwitz DF, Neilson JC. Overall, KL B-1&2 protocol for deference and protocol for relaxation: behavior modification appendix B. In: Horwitz DF, Neilson JC, editors. Clinical behavioral medicine for small animals. St. Louis (MO): Mosby; 1997. p. 410–5.

[16] Sherman CK, Reisner IR, Taliaferro LA, et al. Characteristics, treatment, and outcome of 99 cases of aggression between dogs. Appl Anim Behav Sci 1996;47:91–108.

[17] Pryor PA, Hart BL, Bain MJ, et al. Causes of urine marking in cats and the effects of environmental management on frequency of marking. J Am Vet Med Assoc 2001;219(12): 1709–13.

[18] Denerolle P, White SD, Taylor TS, et al. Organic diseases mimicking acral lick dermatitis in six dogs. J Am Anim Hosp Assoc 2007;43:215–20.

[19] Virga V. Self directed behaviors in dogs and cats. Vet Med 2005;100(3):212–23.

[20] Weisglas SE, Landsberg GM, Yager JA, et al. Underlying medical conditions in cats with presumptive psychogenic alopecia. J AmVet Med Assoc 2006;228(11):1705–9.

Vet Clin Small Anim 38 (2008) 1023–1041

VETERINARY CLINICS
SMALL ANIMAL PRACTICE

ELSEVIER
SAUNDERS

Canine Aggression Toward Unfamiliar People and Dogs

Lore I. Haug, DVM

South Texas Veterinary Behavior Services, 2627 Cordes Drive, Sugar Land, TX 77479, USA

Dog aggression is a serious public health issue in the United States. More than 4 million dog bites to humans are estimated to occur each year [1], and up to 42% of dogs presented to behavior clinics do so for aggression toward other dogs [2]. Aggression places a serious strain on the human–animal bond. Dogs frequently are surrendered to shelters for behavioral reasons, including aggression [3]. Additionally, injuries to victims can result in owners' incurring significant financial and legal burdens. Although aggression is a normal behavior in all animal species, it becomes problematic when it develops in abnormal intensities or contexts, manifests toward aberrant targets (eg, is self-directed), becomes dangerous to other people and animals, and/or interferes with the human–animal bond.

DIAGNOSIS AND CLASSIFICATION

Different authors have classified aggressive behavior in various ways using either functional or categorical divisions. Common categorical terminology can facilitate professional communication; however, such a scheme does not accurately describe all patients—even humans (as evidenced by the number of "disorder unspecified" labels found in the American Psychiatric Association's *Diagnostic and Statistical Manual of Mental Disorders*). In a reductionist sense, canine aggression towards unfamiliar people and dogs generally occurs because of fear, resource guarding (protection of territory, owners, or other animals), or predation. In many cases, dogs present with multiple forms of aggression.

Fear-motivated aggression is the most common diagnosis in dogs aggressive toward unfamiliar stimuli, even when elements of territoriality are present. Offensive posturing by the dog does not rule out anxiety or fear as an underlying cause [4]. The distance to the stimulus and previous learning affect the dog's behavioral presentation. Many dogs show highly offensive posturing when behind a barrier or when the trigger stimulus is far away. As the stimulus approaches or the barrier is removed, the dog's behavior may become more ambiguous and finally reflect outright fear. It is common for dogs to be highly

E-mail address: sykevet@aol.com

0195-5616/08/$ – see front matter
doi:10.1016/j.cvsm.2008.04.005

reactive or aggressive toward other dogs while on leash but then to interact appropriately while off leash. Several theories are postulated to explain this behavior. First, the dog may feel trapped by the confines of the leash, which limits the dog's movements, including its ability to retreat. Second, a tight leash (especially if the owner also is pulling actively) while the dog is approaching or greeting another dog may alter the dog's posture sufficiently to send misleading signals. These signals may trigger the recipient dog to react agonistically, with a scuffle ensuing. Over time, the dog learns that on-leash greetings are unpredictable and potentially dangerous, and the dog becomes preemptively defensive. Third, excitable, but friendly, dogs often are punished with leash corrections for overly exuberant behavior around other dogs. Again, over time the dog learns that the approach of other dogs predicts unpleasant and potentially painful circumstances, generating defensive behavior.

Territorial behavior manifests primarily in the dog's home and yard but also may occur in the car or in areas where the dog is walked habitually. Territorial behavior tends to be most intense directly along the boundary line, and dogs may protect small territories more intensely than large ones [5]. Unlike fear aggression, which often manifests at an early age, territorial and protective behavior are not expected to occur until 6 months of age or older, when the dog approaches social maturity [6]; however, these latter types of aggression frequently have elements of fear as well.

Dogs showing apparent protective behavior more commonly are fear aggressive but become more offensive in the presence of their owner. It is speculated that this change occurs because the owner may have reinforced the dog inadvertently or, alternatively, has punished the dog in the presence of strangers or other dogs, intensifying the dog's emotional reaction to the stimulus. Dominance-related aggression typically is directed toward dogs with which the dog has frequent close, social contact. On occasion, however, dogs do seem to engage in status conflicts with strange people and, more commonly, with unfamiliar dogs. This behavior occurs in relatively close proximity to the stimulus, where postural signaling is most effective; thus dominance probably is not the diagnosis if the dog shows aggressive behavior toward the stimulus from a distance. Predatory reactions are more likely to be directed toward small dogs and fast-moving objects such as joggers and cyclists [7].

ETIOLOGY AND DEVELOPMENT

The development of aggressive behavior frequently is complicated and multifactorial. Problems associated with aggression in dogs fall into two broad categories: (1) normal dogs expressing normal but unacceptable behavior or (2) abnormal dogs reacting out of context to the environment [8]. The boundaries of "normal" behavior are not fixed rigidly: perinatal factors (intrauterine environment, maternal and sibling interactions), experience (socialization and learning), and biologic correlates (genetics, hormones, and neurophysiologic factors) all affect the expression of the behavior.

Genetics and Breed Influences

Selection of phenotypic and behavioral characteristics in dog breeds has resulted in various changes in social competency. Some breeds do show tendencies toward certain forms of aggression [4,9]. Behavioral traits, including aggression, have been identified as clustering in lines or families within a breed [10] or even to be related to coat color patterns [11]. The heritability of owner impressions of aggressive behavior toward dogs and humans in Golden Retrievers has been estimated as high as 81% [12]. A group of studies by Svartberg [13,14] identified consistent heritability of a boldness/shyness personality factor in dogs. Genetics also influences behavior through effects on neurotransmitter systems and other biologic correlates.

Biological Correlates of Aggression

Hormones and gonadectomy

A vast body of literature has examined the effects of sex steroids, particularly testosterone, on aggression in various species. Although testosterone does influence the expression of aggressive behavior, there is a complex interplay between testosterone, social status, neurotransmitters systems, gender, and environmental context [15]. Castration of male dogs affects sexually dimorphic behaviors and will reduce mounting, urine marking, and roaming. Reductions in territoriality and aggression toward other dogs (particularly other males) occurs, but to a lesser degree [9,16,17]. Ovariohysterectomy in females does not influence aggressive behavior significantly or consistently [18]. Kim and colleagues [19] evaluated seven intact and seven ovariohysterectomized German Shepherd bitches for reactivity and aggression and found that 5 months after spaying the spayed bitches showed significantly more reactivity than intact bitches. Gonadectomy should not be expected to play a major role in controlling aggression in dogs.

Neurotransmitters and neural correlates

The biologic basis of aggression is complex. Studies of violence and aggression in humans have focused heavily on the neurotransmitter serotonin (5-HT). The 5-HT system is associated with behavioral inhibition [20]. Evidence links 5-HT deficiency to aggression, but this effect is difficult to isolate from its effects on impulsivity and social behavior, because serotonin also tends to improve both these traits [21]. Reisner and colleagues [22] found lower levels of the serotonin metabolite 5-HIAA in the cerebrospinal fluid of dominant aggressive dogs than in nonaggressive dogs. Other studies of aggressive dogs also have found differences in serotonin receptor densities and function in various brain regions [23]. Biologic correlates may be particularly relevant for the classically "reactive" dog. These dogs respond to even mild or apparently nonthreatening stimuli in a volatile manner, and this reaction may be intensified if the stimulus appears suddenly. Intermittent explosive disorder (IED) in humans may serve as a model for such dogs. Human patients who have IED are defined by impulsive aggressive behavior and are highly reactive to even low-level provocation. These patients rate higher on general anger and hostility than do groups with other psychiatric diagnoses [24]. Patients who have IED also are impaired in their recognition of some facial signals [25], which can affect their social proficiency. Dogs have been shown to have reduced competency in social signaling compared with wolves [18]. Perhaps dogs have deficits in signal interpretation contributing to the comparatively higher level of aggression in dogs than in wolves.

The limbic system, chiefly the amygdala, processes threat and emotional responses. As part of the temporal lobe, the amygdala has a low seizure threshold. Partial seizures in the temporal lobe can trigger feelings of fear, anxiety, irritability, and anger. If a hypersensitivity develops in the amygdala so that a subseizure threshold of neuronal excitability exists, emotional disturbances could arise. This possibility is supported by the fact that human patients who have this behavioral and emotional profile improve when taking anticonvulsant medication [26]. A hyperresponsive amygdala easily could describe the "reactive" dog mentioned previously. Essentially, the amygdala sends a high rate of false alarms that activate the fight–flight system and the regions of the brain responsible for vigilance, attention, anxiety, and fear. Some support for this conjecture comes from studies by Jacobs and colleagues [27] showing that aggressive dogs have higher basolateral nucleus group volumes and neuronal densities in the amygdala than do nonaggressive dogs. Basolateral nucleus groups of aggressive dogs also were shown to have more neurons containing neurokinin 1, which is involved in regulation of aggressive behavior [28]. Furthermore, there are dense concentrations of 5-HT receptors in the amygdala. Serotonin has a net inhibitory effect in the amygdala, so 5-HT–deficient states would result in compromised braking of amygdalar reactions [26].

Perinatal environment and early experience

A puppy's perinatal environment can have a lasting impact on its adult behavior. Maternal stress or early postnatal stress can permanently alter an animal's reactivity to future stress [29,30]. Studies indicate that low-level postnatal stress (brief maternal separation and neonate handling) is protective. It reduces hypothalamic-pituitary-adrenal (HPA) reactivity and increases hippocampal 5-HT. In contrast, more severe stress (prenatal stress, prolonged maternal separation, perinatal illness) can increase the HPA axis responsiveness to physiologic and psychologic insults in the future [29,31]. Therefore, breeders should be counseled carefully on the perinatal environment of their litters.

Socialization deficits are arguably the most prominent factor in the development of aggression in physiologically normal dogs. Unfortunately, the amount of socialization required for optimal development of any individual is unknown. Roll and Unshelm [32] noted that 44% of a population of dog-aggressive dogs had few or no interactions with conspecifics from 5 weeks to 5 months of age. Deficits in social interaction may become more problematic as the animal matures and neophobia and competitive interactions become more salient. Mere exposure to other people and dogs is not sufficient to guarantee adequate social skills. Interactions must be monitored to ensure that the puppy has a positive and enriching experience.

Influence of learning
All forms of aggression are modified by learning. Aggression is about local control of the environment. If an animal learns that aggression will alter the environment in a desirable way, reinforcement occurs, and the animal will show that behavior pattern in a similar circumstance in the future. The power of reinforcement emphasizes the importance of avoiding trigger situations during management and treatment. See the article by Horwitz in this issue for further details.

TREATMENT

In dogs, the origin and progression of aggression to unfamiliar stimuli can vary, as can the associated behavioral presentation. Selecting the most appropriate treatment course depends on the animal's behavioral phenotype and the owner's resources and capabilities. Clinicians should explain each step of the treatment process carefully. Techniques should be demonstrated when appropriate and feasible. Owners must understand that altering the dog's behavior will take time, and improvement may not occur in a linear fashion. Although most owners do not want a lesson in neurophysiology, a brief and simple explanation of the persistence of neural circuits, particularly those associated with fear-related behaviors, can help owners understand their dog's behavioral responses. Setbacks are a typical part of most therapy programs, although the program should be designed and modified periodically to minimize them.

For some owners, the number of environmental changes and interventions can be overwhelming. Breaking the interventions down into progressions will help owners accomplish goals successfully and see more rapid response. This early positive reinforcement for the owner can improve compliance greatly. Treatment programs can be divided into three phases: management, foundation exercises, and stimulus-specific behavior modification exercises.

Management
Environmental management involves addressing the animal's biologic needs and preventing further rehearsal of inappropriate behavior patterns. Safety precautions also must be implemented.

Exercise and enrichment
Many dogs live in environments either grossly deficient in stimulation or replete with inappropriate stimulation. Additionally, as a dog's behavior becomes more problematic, the dog tends to be even more isolated from the environment. Many owners cease walking their dogs altogether, and dogs with territorial behavior often are relegated to spending large amounts of time crated or penned outside. The profound lack of mental and physical exercise compounds the dog's frustration and agitation and decreases the latency to arousal around triggering stimuli. Owners must find ways to exercise their dogs safely. They must walk the dog at times and in places where they are unlikely to encounter other people or dogs, even if the owner must drive the dog to an acceptable area. As well as burning off excess energy, exercise may help by elevating levels

of norepinephrine and 5-HT in the brain and releasing endogenous endorphins [33], the latter two of which have calming and anxiolytic effects [34,35]. Dogs ideally should receive at least 30 continuous minutes of aerobic exercise per day, because research indicates that prolonged aerobic exercise is more effective in triggering opioid-mediated effects on mood and sympathetic activity [36,37].

Mental stimulation through environmental enrichment helps occupy dogs that have limited physical exercise routines and that are left alone for long periods. Enrichment increases behavioral adaptation [31], in part by improving the animal's problem-solving skills. Rotating toys, feeding from food-dispensing devices, and engaging the dog in activities requiring problem solving (eg, training and discrimination tasks) all should be part of the dog's normal routine. Training even simple tricks is excellent mental stimulation and helps strengthen the dog–owner bond as well as increasing the dog's skill set.

Preventing inappropriate behavior
Dogs that have a long-standing history of aggressive behavior have developed a learned, conditioned reaction to trigger stimuli. Accordingly, owners also have become conditioned to anticipate unpleasant encounters. Most aggressive outbursts occur repeatedly in a handful of contexts such that these environments alone can predict the appearance of unfamiliar dogs and people. When the dog and the owner are exposed to these environments, both undergo anticipatory changes in autonomic arousal that push the dog closer to the reactive threshold even in the absence of triggering stimuli [38]. Temporarily removing the dog from these contexts (and from exposure to triggering stimuli) will facilitate the conditioning of more desirable behavioral responses. Avoidance also reduces the risk of injury to other people and dogs. The dog should not be exposed to any such stimuli until later in the rehabilitation process and only during controlled training sessions. For dogs that are aggressive when away from home, exercise modalities and locations must be altered, or the dog must be kept beyond its threshold distance for the stimulus. If the dog is aggressive inside the car, car rides should be minimized or stopped altogether. Some dogs are less reactive if crated while in the car, and the crate can be covered to prevent the dog from seeing stimuli outside. Similarly, inside the house, the dog should be prevented from patrolling windows and doors for passing people or dogs by blocking windows (eg, closing blinds) or gating the dog away from the front of house, especially in the owner's absence. If necessary, the dog can be crated or closed into a room with no or few windows and protected from outside noises. While the owner is home, the dog can be handled more safely and will respond more reliably if fitted with a head collar and dragline, which can be used to interrupt inappropriate behavior immediately but calmly. When visitors arrive, the dog should be confined before the visitor actually enters the house, ideally in an area where the dog cannot see the doorway through which the visitor arrives. If the dog is aggressive only as the visitor enters, but not afterward, the dog can be allowed out of

confinement, under supervision, and on leash with a head collar, once the dog is quiet and the visitor is settled.

Management tools

Helping the owner gain some sense of control over the dog is a valuable step early in a behavior program. Muzzle-loop head collars such as the Gentle Leader (Premier Pet Products, Inc., Richmond, Virginia) (Fig. 1) are especially advantageous for large and/or aggressive dogs. These collars provide excellent control over the dog's head, thereby allowing the owner to manipulate the direction of the dog's focus. Additionally, the owner can close the dog's mouth gently but firmly, which will prevent a bite in an emergency situation and allow humane correction of inappropriate behavior.

Dogs with a previous bite history, with severe or escalating aggression, and/ or with owners that have difficulty controlling them should be trained to wear a muzzle. The muzzle must allow the dog to pant and accept food treats. Provided the dog cannot separate its canine teeth enough to grip another person or dog, a nylon sleeve muzzle can be used as effectively as a basket muzzle. If the muzzle its to be left on for long periods of time, the basket muzzle may be the preferable choice. Both types of muzzles limit panting, and care must be taken when they are used in hot weather. The dog must be adapted to both head collars and muzzles gradually in a manner that associates the devices with pleasant experiences. Neither piece of equipment should ever be placed on the dog as a form of punishment.

Not all dogs can wear a muzzle or head collar because of behavioral, medical, or conformational limitations. Other collar types and harnesses (eg, Easy Walk, Premier Pet Products, Inc.; Zuba Dream Walker, Zuba Pets, Menlo Park, California) are available that may improve the owner's control. Punitive collars such as a prong, slip chain, or electronic stimulation should be avoided. Punitive actions that elevate fear and/or cause the dog pain may be associated

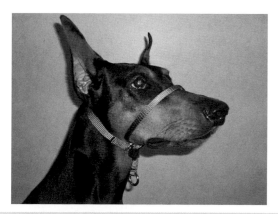

Fig. 1. The Gentle Leader head collar (Premier Pet Products, Inc., Richmond, Virginia).

with the trigger stimulus rather than with the dog's own behavior [39]. This misdirected association is particularly likely if the owner has poor timing and mechanical skills, because the dog will be unable to associate the correction consistently with a specific behavior. This unpredictable punishment actually will increase the dog's anxiety level.

Dogs should be handled on a 4- or 6-foot nylon or leather leash. Retractable leashes are inappropriate and dangerous, because they provide poor control and can cause injury to the owner or the dog if the cord becomes wrapped around part of the body. Cotton long lines can be used to control the dog for exercise purposes, because aggressive dogs should never be off leash in public.

Dogs that are visually reactive may benefit by reducing the clarity of their visual field. The Calming Cap (Premier Pet Products, Inc.) is an elastic, semi-transparent cloth "hood" that covers the dog's eyes. This device can be extremely useful during car rides and also can be used in the home or on walks. TTouch body wraps (Linda Tellington-Jones, Santa Fe, New Mexico) and the Anxiety Wrap (Animals Plus, Huntington, Indiana) have proven effective in calming some excitable or anxious dogs, although no studies have evaluated them in a controlled manner. These products provide tactile pressure over the dog's body for a swaddling or acupressure effect.

Dealing with unplanned exposures

One goal of good management is to reduce uncontrolled stimulus exposures; however, unexpected contacts do occur even with highly dedicated and attentive owners. Owners may carry a pop-open umbrella or Direct Stop citronella spray (Premier Pet Products, Inc.) for dealing with free-ranging dogs. Some dogs can be discouraged with a firm, "No! Go home!" and others may be distracted by throwing a large handful of treats directly at the dog. Well-meaning people should be directed gently but firmly to avoid approaching the dog. Training the dog in advance to perform an emergency U-turn allows calm but rapid escape from a potentially volatile situation. The muzzle-loop head collars permit the owner to control the dog's head and mouth to prevent a bite (to the target or the owner if the dog is prone to redirect) without the need for punitive measures should another person or dog approach too closely.

In a number of cases, alterations in diet and exercise (mental and physical) and reduced exposure to provocative situations improve a dog's behavior sufficiently that the owner is content with management alone. This strategy is a viable one, particularly for time-restricted owners of dog-aggressive dogs, when avoiding contact with other dogs is relatively easy.

Foundation Exercises

The second level of intervention focuses on training foundation exercises, which increase the dog's skill set and give the dog alternative ways to respond to stimuli. The exercises also are designed to amplify the owner's general control over the dog and to improve the dog's focus on and responsiveness to the owner.

Basic cue response

Although many dogs previously were enrolled in a puppy or basic obedience class, an amazingly large number of owners have never sought any type of training for their dogs, even for dogs that have serious behavior issues. Few dogs with aggressive behavior are sufficiently proficient at even basic obedience behaviors. Although obedience itself will not resolve an aggression problem, these cues are important as a way for an owner to request alternative responses from the dog [40]. In situations where the dog is uncertain as to the most appropriate behavioral response, basic behaviors can provide the dog with clarity and safety if the behaviors have been trained previously and practiced in a clear and consistent manner. The goal of training is twofold: (1) to obtain reliable response to the cues, and (2) to condition the dog to become calm and relaxed when performing the behaviors. The latter is crucial and is done by rewarding the dog only for relaxed responses once the dog has a basic understanding of the behavior itself. At a minimum the dog should be able to respond to cues for "sit," "down," "stay," and "come." The dog should be able to walk calmly on leash by the owner's side and also respond to its name by orienting to the owner. Targeting exercises (eg, the dog touching its nose to a target stick or the owner's hand) also are valuable. These behaviors are easy to teach and are easy for the dog to learn, typically resulting in highly reliable behavior. Among other things, targeting can be used to reorient a distracted dog and to lead or lure the dog away from a problematic situation.

All behaviors should be trained using positive reinforcement. Positive reinforcement training establishes a classically conditioned positive emotional response (a "pleasure" feeling) to both the cue and the performance of the behavior. Training based on punishment may be associated with higher levels of behavior problems [41]. The addition of a bridge signal or conditioned reinforcer (eg, clicker, whistle) improves reinforcement clarity and can be used in future exercises as discussed later.

Establishing owner-focused interactions

Leadership programs frequently are recommended to establish command–response interactions between the dog and the owner and stress the importance of interacting with the dog only when the dog is calm. The owner begins to establish consistent behavioral criteria for any interaction with the dog (ie, petting, feeding, starting a training session, putting on the dog's collar, opening doorways). Although it is most important that family members participate in these rules, visitors and other unfamiliar people are encouraged to abide by the protocol as well. Four basic criteria are required of the dog. These criteria can be introduced singly or together, depending on the dog's baseline behavior and the owner's skill:

1. Respond to any requested cue behavior (eg, sit) within an established time frame.
2. Remain calm during the entire interaction.
3. Remain focused on the owner during the interaction. The dog is encouraged to make eye contact and look to the owner rather than focusing on another resource or target.

4. Remain outside a previously designated "personal space" around the owner. This behavior keeps the dog from crowding the owner (eg, to get through a doorway) and also reduces nuisance behaviors such as jumping and mouthing.

The criteria for focus and calmness are by far the most important of the four. In all situations, if the dog fails to maintain an established criterion throughout the interaction, the owner aborts the interaction and directs the dog again. No verbal or physical punishment is applied. Once the dog has attained criterion again, the interaction can resume or start over.

Relaxation Tasks and Safety Cues

Relaxation tasks

Owners of aggressive dogs frequently state that the dog becomes so aroused that the dog is unresponsive in the presence of the triggering stimulus. Owners frequently try to calm or reprimand the dog to halt the aggressive reaction. The flaw in this approach is that such dogs lack emotional control and generally do not know how to relax and self-regulate their arousal, even on a daily basis. Therefore the owner's attempts to calm the dog will be futile. In fact, the owner's mounting tension and frustration typically raises the dog's arousal even further. Relaxation must be taught to the dog in a methodical manner in an environment initially free of distraction.

Structured down-stay (or sit-stay) exercises should be practiced as a baseline relaxation task [42]. The dog is trained to maintain a short, relaxed down-stay and then gradually is exposed to increasing levels of generic environmental distractions and human activities. To further increase the dog's baseline relaxation, behaviors that a dog exhibits voluntarily when normally relaxed can be reinforced and placed on cue. Because the dog already is inclined to perform these behaviors, they are relatively easy to put under stimulus control. Canine massage and TTouch also are excellent exercises to establish changes in relaxation in association with a safety signal. Voluntary lateral recumbency is associated with relaxation in dogs. This "play dead" behavior (Fig. 2) can be placed on cue to allow the owner another tool for lowering arousal in the face of a provocative stimulus. Because this position is highly vulnerable for the dog, it is imperative that the dog never be physically forced into this position, either during the training phase or during a real situation. If the dog will not perform the behavior when cued, the behavior either is not sufficiently rehearsed or the dog has been placed in a situation that is too stressful for its stage of training. Forcing the dog into this position will seriously erode the dog's trust in the handler (Relaxation tasks should serve as another form of safety signal.) The effectiveness of these behaviors can be enhanced by augmenting them with other safety signals such as conditioned odors or having the dog perform them on a "relaxation rug," which can be transported to various locations.

All exercises are trained first within the owner's home in a quiet environment. Once the dog is proficient, the tasks are repeated in other areas both on and off the owner's property. The dog never should be asked to perform

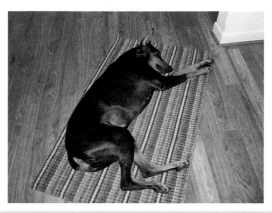

Fig. 2. The lateral recumbency ("play dead") position is used as a relaxation task. This dog has learned to perform this behavior reliably even in the presence of some fear-inducing distractions, and obeying this command helps control her arousal. Relaxation is shaped during the training of the behavior; however, note the tucking of the dog's tail and the slight flexion of the right hind leg up toward the dog's body. These signs indicate that shaping for further relaxation is needed.

in an environment that it is not yet ready to handle. Asking the dog to hold a relaxation position when it is in a stressful environment will erode the value of the behavior as a safety cue.

Safety cues and signals
Animals readily make associations between contextual (environmental) stimuli and emotional experiences that occur when those stimuli are present. For example, a dog in a veterinary examination room receiving a painful injection while resting on a blue rug may become afraid of blue rugs. Even though the rug was neutral and did not harm the dog, the rug became associated with the context in which the dog was hurt or frightened. Through a similar learning process, a dog can associate environmental stimuli with pleasant, safe experiences.

Safety signals are environmental stimuli that become paired with relaxed physiologic states in safe environments. Safety signals can be tactile, olfactory, visual, or auditory. They also can be previously trained behaviors (cues). The stimuli themselves eventually generate a relaxed state in the dog when the animal is exposed to them. Exercises addressing stimulus-specific responses revolve primarily around classical conditioning paradigms such as counterconditioning. Classical conditioning is a powerful tool for establishing baseline changes in physiologic and psychologic relaxation and in establishing the safety signals used during the last phase of training.

Conditioning safety cues involves choosing a specific stimulus (eg, a specific dog bed, small rug, or odor) and pairing its presence with pleasant activities and the relaxation tasks. For instance, the dog can be cued to lie on the dog bed and then rewarded when it does so in a relaxed manner. During the conditioning process, the dog is never asked to lie on the bed when it is agitated, as a punishment, or while anything unpleasant to the dog (eg, nail trimming) is being performed. With repetitions the dog becomes conditioned to relax when asked to lie on the bed or when other safety cues are present.

Safety cues should be portable and easy to reproduce but also fairly unique to the environment in which they eventually will be used (eg, out on walks, at the veterinary clinic, when visitors come to the house). This specificity prevents the dog from habituating to their presence in the environment. The dog should be exposed to the safety signal only during conditioning sessions to ensure that the pairing of cue and relaxation remains as consistent as possible.

Stimulus-Specific Behavior Modification Exercises

Stimulus-specific exercises center on desensitization-counterconditioning (DCC) drills. Typical methodology has both classical and operant conditioning components, although variations may focus heavily on one element over the other. In traditional DCC, the animal is exposed to a low-level stimulus, and the presence of the stimulus is paired with something the dog finds rewarding, such as food or play. The previously described down-stay relaxation task serves as the foundation for stimulus-specific DCC. The trigger stimulus becomes a new distraction added to the protocol. The dog is asked to sit or down-stay, preferably in the presence of a previously established safety signal, and then the dog is exposed to a low-level stimulus (eg, a dog or person) at a distance such that the dog briefly alerts but then returns focus to the owner. If the dog reacts to the stimulus, the stimulus is too close or too intense. The dog then is rewarded for remaining calm in the cued position.

For each stimulus category (eg, dogs or people), the owner should develop a hierarchical list with the stimulus composition least likely to arouse the dog at the top and the stimulus composition most likely to trigger arousal at the bottom. The more intermediary stimuli listed, the better. The owner also should determine the thresholds at which the dog (1) alerts/orients to the stimulus, (2) barks/growls, and (3) lunges or tries to bite. This list becomes the dog's general training syllabus.

DCC sessions are divided into four base criteria: distance (between the dog and the trigger stimulus), duration (that the dog is exposed to the stimulus during any one trial), intensity (of the behavior or physical characteristics of the stimulus), and number (of stimuli present at one time during the trial). During any one trial, only one criterion should be manipulated. For example, if an owner finishes a trial with a child 30 feet away from the dog, on the next trial the child should not move closer to the dog and change his/her behavior. Rather, the child either should be asked to move closer or to alter his/her behavior. Once the dog can master each criterion individually, sessions can begin to incorporate multiple criteria at one time.

Highly aroused dogs may benefit from beginning DCC with audiotapes of sounds associated with the trigger stimulus (eg, dog tags, barking, footsteps on the sidewalk, human voices). This technique allows the owner to begin the process in the safety of the dog's home. For dogs with territorial aggression, sessions should include sounds of doorbells and knocking. The dog also should be trained to sit or lie calmly away from the door when the door is opened and someone enters. This behavior is accomplished first with family members, then with familiar visitors, and finally progresses to unfamiliar visitors.

Some dogs are so reactive that any visual exposure results in a dramatic aggressive display even if the stimulus is hundreds of yards away. For these dogs, a purely classical conditioning paradigm using a previously conditioned bridge stimulus (ie, clicker or whistle) may be more appropriate initially. The dog is placed in a sit-stay position and is controlled by a head collar. The stimulus (eg, a person) steps into view from behind a solid barrier at a great distance for only 1 or 2 seconds before stepping back behind the barrier. (This brief appearance reduces the likelihood that the dog's arousal will continue to escalate.) As the person comes into view, the owner immediately applies the bridge stimulus, irrespective of the dog's behavior, and then offers the dog food or a toy. The dog may be so aroused by the sight of the person that it refuses the food. In the absence of the bridge signal, this level of arousal means conditioning may not occur, because the dog may refuse the food or toy. The bridge signal allows the beginning of conditioning even if the dog refuses to eat the food or play with the toy. The dog is allowed to return to baseline arousal before the process is repeated. Over time, this method can establish an "auto-look" to the owner after the person comes into view. This looking to the owner is the beginning of a threshold, in that there is a brief period of nonreaction. At this point traditional DCC can begin.

Diet and Nutrition

There is considerable controversy and conflicting data on the influence of dietary factors on aggressive behavior. Few controlled studies have evaluated nutritional effects in dogs. Dodman and colleagues [43] evaluated the influence of dietary protein level on aggressive behavior and found that reductions in protein may help reduce territorial behavior associated with fear, but the effect was not robust, and the diet did not affect other types of aggression studied. Studies in humans have shown changes in aggression and violence with dietary tryptophan supplementation [44] and one study indicated a possible effect in dogs [45]. Anecdotal reports indicate possible benefits of raw food diets, grain-free diets, and low-protein diets; however, no controlled studies have been done with the former two diets. How any individual animal responds to dietary change is unknown and seems to be a matter of trial and error. Gesch and colleagues [46] noted improvements in violence and antisocial behavior in prisoners receiving a supplemental vitamin-mineral and fatty acid preparation. Similar results might be obtainable in dogs.

Pheromone and Aromatherapy

The canine olfactory system is well developed and represents a significant portion of the dog's brain mass. The olfactory system is highly connected to the limbic system. Dogs have a functional vomeronasal organ that transmits information to the accessory olfactory bulb and then on to the amygdala [47]. Olfactory stimuli can play a substantial role in the development and resolution of behavior issues. Dog-appeasing pheromone (DAP; Ceva Santé Animale, Libourne, Gironde, France) is a synthetic analogue of the pheromone secreted by lactating bitches. Recent studies have shown merit in its use for increasing adaptability in newly adopted puppies [48], for improving performance in puppies attending puppy classes [49], for reducing signs of fear or anxiety in veterinary settings [50], and for treating fear of fireworks [51]. Wells [52] has demonstrated that lavender scent can reduce excitability during car rides, and it also increases relaxation in shelter settings [53]. Lavender can be used spontaneously or conditioned as a safety cue to be used in the home or applied to a bandana the dog wears while away from home.

Pharmacologic Intervention

Currently there are no medications labeled for treating aggression disorders in dogs. There are few controlled clinical studies evaluating drug therapy in aggressive dogs. Virga and colleagues [54] found no benefit with amitriptyline use in aggressive dogs as compared with behavior modification alone. White and colleagues [55] also found no effect beyond placebo in the use of clomipramine for dominance-related aggression. One study evaluating the use of fluoxetine in dogs with dominance-related aggression did find a small effect, but the improvement also could be attributed to placebo effects [56].

Despite the lack of data supporting clinical efficacy, anecdotal reports indicate that pharmacologic intervention can facilitate or expedite behavior therapy in some cases. Benefit may be most likely if (1) the aggression is related to high-anxiety states or fearful behavior, (2) the animal appears to have a concurrent impulse-control disorder, or (3) the dog is truly "reactive," that is, the behavioral profile supports the possibility of amygdalar hyperreactivity.

Selective serotonin reuptake inhibitors (SSRIs) manipulate serotonin concentration in the synaptic cleft, and their effect is relatively specific for serotonin. They have antidepressant, anxiolytic, and anticompulsive effects [57]. SSRIs currently are the primary class prescribed for aggression problems in dogs (Table 1). Fluoxetine, recently approved for use in dogs for separation anxiety under the name Reconcile (Eli Lilly, Indianapolis, Indiana), is the SSRI with the longest history of use for behavior problems in dogs. Its use for aggression is extra-label. All SSRIs require continuous prolonged administration to produce therapeutic changes. Fluoxetine typically is well tolerated; however, reported side effects include sedation, gastrointestinal upset, anorexia, irritability, agitation, and seizures [58]. Fluoxetine and paroxetine [59] inhibit various cytochrome P-450 enzymes; therefore, potential drug interactions should be monitored carefully. Other commonly used SSRIs include paroxetine,

Table 1
Dosages for common psychotherapeutic agents in dogs

Drug	Dosage	Reference
Azaspirone		
Buspirone	1.0–2 mg/kg every 8–12 hours	
Anticonvulsants		
Carbamazepine	4–8 mg/kg every 12 hours	
Gabapentin	10–30 mg/kg every 8–12 hours	Plumb [66]
Beta-blockers		
Pindolol	0.125–0. 25 mg/kg every 12–24 hours	Plumb [66]
Propranolol	5–40 mg/dog every 8 hours	Plumb [66]
Benzodiazepine		
Alprazolam	0.02–0.1 mg/kg every 8–12 hours	
Clorazepate	2 mg/kg every 12 hours	
Diazepam	0.55–2.2 mg/kg every 8–12 hours	
Selective serotonin reuptake inhibitors		
Citalopram	0.5–1.0 mg/kg every 24 hrs	
Fluoxetine	1.0–2.0 mg/kg every 24 hours	
Paroxetine	0.5–1.5 mg/kg every 24 hours	
Sertraline	0.5–4.0 mg/kg every 24 hours	
Tricyclic antidepressants		
Amitriptyline	1.0–4.0 mg/kg every 12 hours	
Clomipramine	1.0–3.0 mg/kg every 12 hours	

Data from Crowell-Davis SL, Murray T, Seibert LM. Veterinary psychopharmacology. Ames (IA): Blackwell Publishing; 2006; and Simpson BS, Papich MG. Pharmacologic management in veterinary behavioral medicine. Vet Clin North Am Small Anim Pract 2003;33(2):365–404, unless otherwise noted.

sertraline, fluvoxamine, and citalopram. Sertraline and fluoxetine often are useful choices for older dogs because they do not have the anticholinergic effects of paroxetine that may interfere with cognitive function [60].

Tricyclic antidepressants (TCAs) also have a long history of use for behavior problems in dogs. Amitriptyline and clomipramine (labeled for separation anxiety in dogs under the name Clomicalm [Novartis Animal Health, Greensboro, North Carolina]) are the two most frequently prescribed. These drugs have both serotonin and norepinephrine reuptake properties, with clomipramine being more specific for serotonin [60]. TCAs also have anticholinergic, antihistaminic, and alpha-adrenergic blockage effects, which are responsible for most of the observed side effects and can include sedation, constipation, urinary retention, vomiting, diarrhea, agitation, hypotension, and lowered seizure threshold [61].

TCAs seem to be more effective for anxiety- and fear-related disorders. Given the lack of therapeutic effect in the few studies evaluating TCAs for aggression, it might be wiser to reserve these drugs for use in dogs that have concurrent severe anxiety disorders or in cases in which SSRIs have failed to produce any therapeutic response.

Although not commonly used, anticonvulsants such as carbamazepine or gabapentin may have some utility in dogs that seem to have amygdalar hyperreactivity [58]. These drugs sometimes are used in conjunction with SSRIs to control explosive aggression. Buspirone, an azaspirone, is a presynaptic 5-HT1A agonist. It also has partial agonist properties at postsynaptic 5-HT1A receptors. Buspirone has been used to control mild anxiety disorders and generalized anxiety [58]. Its effect on aggressive behavior has not been evaluated, but clinical experience indicates that as a sole therapy it has little role in controlling aggression in dogs.

Serotonin modulators, discussed previously, all require continuous administration for therapeutic effects. Some drugs can be used on a situational basis to control anxiety and frustration that may contribute to aggressive responses. These medications can be given on an as-needed basis, for example, before outings during which avoidance of problematic stimuli is impossible or to enhance success during a controlled training situation. Situational drugs include opioids, beta-blockers, and benzodiazepines. As mentioned previously, opioids can modulate serotonergic transmission and sympathetic activation, thereby reducing heart rate, blood pressure, and anxiety [36]. Similarly beta-blockers have been postulated to reduce anxiety by controlling heart rate changes associated with anxiety, although some beta-blockers (eg, pindolol) have direct serotonergic actions as well. Benzodiazepines are very effective for reducing anxiety, but they also may produce disinhibition of aggression [62,63], particularly in an animal that is highly offensive. Therefore, their use probably should be restricted to animals whose aggression is purely defensive.

There also is little evidence that most natural therapeutics are useful in the treatment of aggression, except for tryptophan, as mentioned earlier, and a milk hydrolyzate, alpha-casozepine, which seems to be beneficial in reducing some forms of anxiety [64]. Crowell-Davis and colleagues [65] provide a more detailed review of medications and their usage in veterinary psychopharmacology.

SUMMARY

Canine aggression toward unfamiliar people and dogs is a common behavior problem. Although a variety of factors are involved in the development of this problem, genetics and socialization deficits play a major role. This problem typically can be well controlled with targeted changes in the animal's environment, implementation of appropriate behavior modification exercises, and adjunctive pharmacologic support where indicated. Owners should be encouraged to seek professional help early in the problem before the dog actually injures another animal or human.

References
[1] Overall K, Love M. Dog bites to humans—demography, epidemiology, injury, and risk. J Am Vet Med Assoc 2001;218(12):1923–34.
[2] Sherman CK, Reisner I, Taliaferro L, et al. Characteristics, treatment, and outcome of 99 cases of aggression between dogs. Appl Anim Behav Sci 1996;47:91–108.
[3] Miller DD, Staats SR, Partlo C, et al. Factors associated with the decision to surrender a pet to an animal shelter. J Am Vet Med Assoc 1996;209(4):738–42.

[4] Lindsay S. Aggressive behavior: basic concepts and principles. In: Handbook of applied dog behavior and training. Etiology and assessment of behavior problems, vol. 2. Ames (IA): Iowa State University Press; 2001. p. 161–201.

[5] Overall K. Canine aggression. In: Clinical behavioral medicine for small animals. St. Louis (MO): Mosby; 1997. p. 88–137.

[6] Reisner I. Differential diagnosis and management of human-directed aggression in dogs. Vet Clin North Am Small Anim Pract 2003;33(2):303–20.

[7] Bowen J. Miscellaneous behaviour problems. In: Horwitz DF, Mills DS, Heath S, editors. BSAVA manual of canine and feline behavioural medicine. Quedgeley, Gloucester (UK): British Small Animal Veterinary Association; 2002. p. 119–27.

[8] Hart B, Hart LA, Bain MJ. General approaches to behavioral pharmacology. In: Canine and feline behavior therapy. Ames (IA): Blackwell Publishing; 2006. p. 63–73.

[9] Hart B, Hart LA, Bain MJ. Aggression toward people. In: Canine and feline behavior therapy. Ames (IA): Blackwell Publishing; 2006. p. 103–28.

[10] Reisner I, Houpt K, Shofer FS. National survey of owner-directed aggression in English Springer Spaniels. J Am Vet Med Assoc 2005;227(10):1594–603.

[11] Podberscek AL, Serpell J. The English Cocker Spaniel: preliminary findings on aggressive behaviour. Appl Anim Behav Sci 1996;47:75–89.

[12] Liinamo A-E, van den Berg L, Leegwater PAJ, et al. Genetic variation in aggression-related traits in Golden Retriever dogs. Appl Anim Behav Sci 2007;104:95–106.

[13] Svartberg K. A comparison of behaviour in test and in everyday life: evidence of three consistent boldness-related personality traits in dogs. Appl Anim Behav Sci 2005;91:103–28.

[14] Svartberg K, Tapper I, Temrin H, et al. Consistency of personality traits in dogs. Anim Behav 2005;69:283–91.

[15] Haug LI. Androgens and 5-HIAA in dogs with intraspecific aggression [master's thesis]. College Station (TX): Texas A&M University; 2003.

[16] Hart B, Hart LA, Bain MJ. Canine and feline behavior therapy. 2nd edition. Ames (IA): Blackwell Publishing; 2006.

[17] Neilson J, Eckstein R, Hart B. Effects of castration on problem behaviors in male dogs with reference to age and duration of behavior. J Am Vet Med Assoc 1997;211(2):180–2.

[18] Mertens P. Canine aggression. In: Horwitz DF, Mills DS, Heath S, editors. BSAVA manual of canine and feline behavioural medicine. Quedgeley, Gloucester (UK): British Small Animal Veterinary Association; 2002. p. 195–215.

[19] Kim HH, Yeon SC, Houpt K, et al. Effects of overiohysterectomy on reactivity in German Shepherd dogs. Vet J 2006;172:154–9.

[20] Hashimoto S, Inoue T, Koyama T. Effects of conditioned fear stress on serotonin neurotransmission and freezing behavior in rats. Eur J Pharmacol 1999;378:23–30.

[21] Higley JD, King ST, Hasert MF, et al. Stability of interindividual differences in serotonin function and its relationship to severe aggression and competent social behavior in Rhesus Macaque females. Neuropsychopharmacology 1996;14:67–76.

[22] Reisner I, Mann JJ, Stanley M, et al. Comparison of cerebrospinal fluid monoamine metabolite levels in dominant-aggressive and non-aggressive dogs. Brain Res 1996;714:57–64.

[23] Badino P, Odore R, Osella MC, et al. Modifications of serotonergic and adrenergic receptor concentrations in the brain of aggressive Canis familiaris. Comp Biochem Physiol A Mol Integr Physiol 2004;139:343–50.

[24] McCloskey MS, Berman ME, Noblett KL, et al. Intermittent explosive disorder-integrated research diagnostic criteria: convergent and discriminant validity. J Psychiatr Res 2006;40:231–42.

[25] Best M, Williams JM, Coccaro EF. Evidence for dysfunctional prefrontal circuit in patients with an impulsive aggressive disorder. Proc Natl Acad Sci U S A 2002;99(12):8448–53.

[26] Keele NB. The role of serotonin in impulsive and aggressive behaviors associated with epilepsy-like neuronal hyperexcitability in the amygdala. Epilepsy Behav 2005;7:325–35.

[27] Jacobs C, Van Den Broeck W, Simoens P. Increased volume and neuronal number of the basolateral nuclear group of the amygdaloid body in aggressive dogs. Brain Res 2006;170(1):119–25.

[28] Jacobs C, Van Den Broeck W, Simoens P. Neurokinin-1 receptor in the basolateral nuclear group of the canine amygdala—comparative study in normal and aggressive dogs. Brain Res 2006;1098(1):106–12.

[29] Sanchez MM, Ladd CO, Plotsky PM. Early adverse experience as a developmental risk factor for later psychopathology: evidence from rodent and primate models. Dev Psychopathol 2001;13:419–49.

[30] Chapillon P, Patin V, Roy V, et al. Effects of pre- and postnatal stimulation on development, emotional, and cognitive aspects in rodents: a review. Dev Psychobiol 2002;41:373–87.

[31] Anisman H, Zaharia MD, Meaney MJ, et al. Do early-life events permanently alter behavioral and hormonal responses to stressors? Int J Dev Neurosci 1998;16(3/4):149–64.

[32] Roll A, Unshelm J. Aggressive conflicts amongst dogs and factors affecting them. Appl Anim Behav Sci 1997;52:229–42.

[33] Lindsay S. Neurobiology of behavior and learning. In: Handbook of applied dog behavior and trainingAdaptation and learning, vol. 1. Ames (IA): Iowa State University Press; 2000. p. 73–126.

[34] Guszkowska M. Effects of exercise an anxiety, depression and mood. Psychiatr Pol 2004;38(4):611–20.

[35] Hebb AL, Poulin JF, Roach SP, et al. Cholecystokinin and endogenous opioid peptides: interactive influence on pain, cognition, and emotion. Prog Neuropsychopharmacol Biol Psychiatry 2005;29(8):1225–38.

[36] Thoren P, Floras JS, Hoffman P, et al. Endorphins and exercise: physiological mechanisms and clinical implications. Med Sci Sports Exerc 1990;22(4):417–28.

[37] Hoffman MD, Shepanski MA, Ruble SB, et al. Intensity and duration threshold for aerobic exercise-induced analgesia to pressure pain. Arch Phys Med Rehabil 2004;85:1183–7.

[38] Lindsay S. Neurobiology and development of aggression. In: Handbook of applied dog behavior and training. Procedures and protocols, vol. 3. Ames (IA): Blackwell Publishing; 2005. p. 279–345.

[39] Lindsay S. Impulsive, extrafamilial, and intraspecific aggression. In: Handbook of applied dog behavior and trainingProcedures and protocols, vol. 3. Ames (IA): Blackwell Publishing; 2005. p. 433–555.

[40] Clark GI, Boyer WN. The effects of dog obedience training and behavioral counseling upon the human-canine relationship. Appl Anim Behav Sci 1993;37:147–59.

[41] Kabaila A. The effects of current training techniques and environmental factors on dog behavior. Anim Welf Sci Ess 2004.

[42] Overall K. Treatment of behavioral problems. In: Clinical behavioral medicine for small animals. St. Louis (MO): Mosby; 1997. p. 274–92.

[43] Dodman N, Reisner I, Shuster L, et al. Effect of dietary protein content on behavior in dogs. J Am Vet Med Assoc 1996;208(3):376–9.

[44] Bjork JM, Doughtery DM, Moeller G, et al. Differential behavioral effects of plasma tryptophan depletion and loading in aggressive and nonaggressive men. Neuropsychopharmacology 2000;22:357–69.

[45] DeNapoli JS, Dodman N, Shuster L, et al. Effect of dietary protein content and tryptophan supplementation on dominance aggression, territorial aggression, and hyperactivity in dogs. J Am Vet Med Assoc 2000;217(4):504–8.

[46] Gesch CB, Hammond SM, Hampson SE, et al. Influence of supplementary vitamins, minerals and essential fatty acids on the antisocial behavior of young adult prisoners. Br J Psychiatry 2002;181:22–8.

[47] Pageat P, Gaultier E. Current research in canine and feline pheromones. Vet Clin North Am Small Anim Pract 2003;33(2):187–211.

[48] Gaultier E, Bonnafous L, Vienet-Legue D, et al. Efficacy of dog appeasing pheromone in reducing stress related behaviors of newly adopted puppies coming from a pet shop. Presented at the American College of Veterinary Behaviorists/American Veterinary Society of Animal Behavior Scientific Paper Session, Washington, DC, July 16, 2007.

[49] Denenberg S, Landsberg G. Evaluation of the effect of dog appeasing pheromones on the reduction of anxiety and fear in puppies during training. Presented at the American College of Veterinary Behaviorists/American Veterinary Society of Animal Behavior Scientific Paper Session, 3–4. Washington, DC, July 16, 2007.

[50] Mills DS, Ramos D, Estelles MG, et al. A triple blind placebo-controlled investigation into the assessment of the effect of dog appeasing pheromone (DAP) on anxiety related behaviour of problem dogs in the veterinary clinic. Appl Anim Behav Sci 2006;98:114–26.

[51] Sheppared G, Mills DS. Evaluation of dog-appeasing pheromone as a potential treatment for dogs fearful of fireworks. Vet Rec 2003;152(14):432–6.

[52] Wells DL. Aromatherapy for travel-induced excitement in dogs. J Am Vet Med Assoc 2006;229(6):964–7.

[53] Graham L, Wells DL, Hepper PG. The influence of olfactory stimulation on the behaviour of dogs housed in a rescue shelter. Appl Anim Behav Sci 2005;91:143–53.

[54] Virga V, Houpt K, Scarlett JM. Efficacy of amitriptyline as a pharmacological adjunct to behavior modification in the management of aggressive behaviors in dogs. J Am Anim Hosp Assoc 2001;37:325–30.

[55] White MM, Neilson J, Hart B. Dominance-related aggression in dogs: effects of treatment with placebo or clomipramine. Presented at American Veterinary Society of Animal Behavior, New Orleans, LA, July 11, 1999.

[56] Dodman N, Donnelly R, Shuster L, et al. Use of fluoxetine to treat dominance aggression in dogs. J Am Vet Med Assoc 1996;209(9):1585–7.

[57] Crowell-Davis SL, Murray T. Selective serotonin reuptake inhibitors. In: Veterinary psychopharmacology. Ames (IA): Blackwell Publishing; 2006. p. 80–110.

[58] Simpson BS, Papich MG. Pharmacologic management in veterinary behavioral medicine. Vet Clin North Am Small Anim Pract 2003;33(2):365–404.

[59] Bourin M, Chue P, Guillon Y. Paroxetine: a review. CNS Drug Rev 2001;7(1):25–47.

[60] Stahl SM. Classical antidepressants, serotonin selective reuptake inhibitors, and noradrenergic reuptake inhibitors. In: Essential psychopharmacology: neuroscientific basis and practical applications. Cambridge (MA): Cambridge University Press; 2000. p. 199–244.

[61] Crowell-Davis SL, Murray T. Tricyclic antidepressants. In: Veterinary psychopharmacology. Ames (IA): Blackwell Publishing; 2006. p. 179–206.

[62] Ben-Porath DD, Taylor SP. The effects of diazepam (Valium) and aggressive disposition on human aggression: an experimental investigation. Addict Behav 2002;27:167–77.

[63] Bond A, Curran HV, Bruce MS, et al. Behavioural aggression in panic disorder after 8 weeks' treatment with alprazolam. J Affect Disord 1995;35:117–23.

[64] Beata C, Beaumon-Graff E, Diaz C, et al. Effects of alpha-casozepine (Zylkene) versus selegiline hydrochloride (Selgian, Anipryl) on anxiety disorders in dogs. J Vet Behav 2007;2(5):175–83.

[65] Crowell-Davis SL, Murray T, Seibert LM. Veterinary psychopharmacology. Ames (IA): Blackwell Publishing; 2006.

[66] Plumb DC. Veterinary drug handbook. 5th edition. Ames (IA): Blackwell Publishing; 2005.

Vet Clin Small Anim 38 (2008) 1043–1063

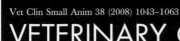
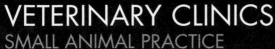

VETERINARY CLINICS
SMALL ANIMAL PRACTICE

Expanding Families: Preparing for and Introducing Dogs and Cats to Infants, Children, and New Pets

Laurie Bergman, VMD[a],*, Lori Gaskins, DVM[b]

[a]Metropolitan Veterinary Associates, 2626 Van Buren Avenue, Norristown, PA 19403, USA
[b]St. Matthew's University School of Veterinary Medicine, P.O. Box 32330 SMB, Grand Cayman KY1-1209, Cayman Islands, BWI

PETS AND THE FAMILY—NEW INTRODUCTIONS

Veterinarians can help clients successfully integrate new members into the family, whether children or additional pets, by ensuring that pet owners see them as a valuable resource for behavioral, as well as medical, concerns. All too often, clients turn to lay sources, such as the Internet or friends, for behavioral assistance [1]. Providing client education material in the hospital will remind clients that veterinarians are the educated professionals to whom they should turn for help in this area. Educating clients about pets' body language during routine appointments and by books or posters in the examination room will help owners understand their pets better. One should inquire about the patient's behavior during all non-emergency appointments, either verbally or through simple questionnaires. Questions in the behavioral history should include the pet's exposure to and reactions to infants, children of different ages, and other animals. This information provides a baseline for the pet's behavior, keeps the behavioral history current regarding family dynamics, and makes it easier for the veterinarian to raise concerns about a patient's behavior [2]. For example, recent research has shown that 77% of dogs presented to a veterinary behavior clinic with a history of biting children also had a history of separation- and/or noise-related anxiety. Knowledge of these seemingly unrelated behavioral problems can help veterinarian make appropriate recommendations to clients who are adding children to their households [3].

When dealing with expanding families, the axiom "an ounce of prevention is worth a pound of cure" rings true. Preparing the existing household pets for the arrival of newcomers can avoid heartbreaking and potentially life-threatening problems [2,4]. Because veterinarians may not always know when a client is planning an addition to the family, outreach to clients and other members of the community can educate pet owners regarding the steps they should take

*Corresponding author. E-mail address: lbergman@alum.barnard.edu (L. Bergman).

0195-5616/08/$ – see front matter
doi:10.1016/j.cvsm.2008.04.004

in advance to help ease the transition and avoid problems. Outreach in the form of announcements in clinic newsletters or local newspapers can alert pet owners that "Preparing the Pets" appointments are available for expectant parents and blended families. Basic information about preparing pets for the arrival of an infant and making the initial introductions can be conveyed through classes offered through local human hospitals or obstetricians. Similar methods can be used to publicize the availability of veterinary assistance in selecting and introducing additional animals to the household. These approaches reach beyond a clinic's existing clientele.

Part of a "Preparing the Pets" appointment is a thorough physical examination to ensure that pets are physically and behaviorally healthy before attempting an introduction to new family members. Irritable aggression in pets results because they are less tolerant of things when ill or stressed, and they can become aggressive if forced to interact when ill [5,6] (see the article by Siebert and Landsberg in this issue). Practitioners or their staff should take time during this appointment to educate owners about canine and feline body language. The goal should be to ensure that clients can recognize signs that a pet is anxious or uncomfortable with a situation. Visual aids such as body-language diagrams [7,8] are very useful (see the article by Levine in this issue for more details). For adults and older children, a board game has been developed that teaches canine body language [9].

The use of pheromones such as dog-appeasing pheromone (DAP, Ceva Santé Animale, Libourne, Cedex, France) or Feliway (Ceva) may help during introductions [10,11] and can be recommended as part of general preparations. Chamomile and aromatherapy with lavender also have been recommended during new pet introductions [12]. These nonprescription treatments have few adverse side effects and are readily available to most pet owners. Veterinarians should be involved in discussing the risks and benefits of these adjunct therapies with their clients, however.

SKILLS FOR LIVING WITH OTHERS

When collecting baseline behavioral information about patients, veterinarians should inquire about the pet's "skills for living with others." These are behaviors or husbandry techniques that pets should be accustomed to well in advance of the arrival of any new addition to the family. Prior planning will reduce the stress on clients and their pets. Training pets to be comfortable with these behaviors will serve as insurance for future family expansions as well as help manage other common situations. Ideally, these topics are discussed with all new puppy and kitten owners and are part of routine preventative health care for adult pets.

Positive Reinforcement Training, Desensitization Instead of Punishment

These techniques are the foundation for the skills the pet will need to live with new additions to the family. Positive reinforcement training is humane, effective, and strengthens the human–animal bond [13]. Rewards are given for good behavior such as following commands and showing relaxed behavior. For example, a dog that excitedly jumps on visitors is taught to sit on command and is rewarded for doing so with treats and petting. He then is kept on leash for added control when greeting people. If he does not sit, he is moved away from the visitors, thus losing the chance for a treat and petting, until he is calm enough to behave properly. Removing the dog is an example of negative punishment, which means that the consequence of misbehavior is the removal of something rewarding (opportunity for petting) to decrease a behavior (jumping). Unlike other types of punishments or reprimands, negative punishment is rarely counterproductive, especially when dealing with anxious animals.

The basic principle of desensitization is used both in teaching new behaviors and in correcting behavior problems. Desensitization involves introducing the new behavior at a level of difficulty that the animal can handle emotionally and gradually increasing the difficulty. For instance, to teach a dog to sit calmly when letting guests into the house, one should start teaching a calm "sit-stay" without people knocking at the door or entering the house and in a location where the pet is completely comfortable. As the dog becomes better at sitting calmly, the steps of a guest knocking at the door and being invited into the house are introduced slowly over multiple training sessions until the dog is able to stay seated through an actual visitor's arrival. By gradually increasing the difficulty of the behavior requested, whether it is teaching the dog to stay in a "down" position for a full minute or helping it overcome its fear of the sound of a crying child, the dog is set up for success. An added benefit of this type of training is that it sets a wonderful example for children to follow as they grow up and interact with pets and other people [14,15]. In addition to being more humane than training through coercive or force-based methods, reward-based training also is safer. Although an adult may be able to administer a choke chain or physical correction correctly, it is unlikely that a child could do so, because of the lack of the strength required and lack of the appropriate timing. The inappropriate use of physical punishment can lead to increased anxiety and aggression [16,17]. Sometimes even a seemingly benign verbal correction, when delivered by a child about whom the pet may be anxious, can lead to defensive aggression (Gary Landsberg, DVM, personal communication 2007). If clients are reluctant to change their training style, the American Veterinary Society of Animal Behavior has excellent information on its website [18] explaining the difficulties and possible adverse effects of using punishment in training and behavior modification.

Space and Separation

The two topics of space and separation go together well, because pets should have comfortable resting areas where they can choose to retreat from interactions, and owners should have the ability to separate their pets physically from people or other animals in the house if needed [2]. The place where a pet chooses to relax on its own may be the place where the owners confine the animal, or it may be a different location. For example, a dog may have a dog bed in the middle of a family room where it rests when the owners are relaxing in the evenings, but it may be confined to the laundry room if physical separation is needed. For cats, the idea of a comfortable resting place can be expanded to include the concept of a "house of plenty." (Leslie Larson Cooper, DVM, personal communication, 2000). This concept involves providing the cat (or cats) with an excess of valuable resources, such as resting areas, hiding places, litter boxes, toys, food, and water dishes. A cat that is uncomfortable with a situation, whether the introduction of a new person or cat to the home or a noisy vacuum cleaner, has the ability to access the things it needs and still avoid the situation that is making it uncomfortable. This provision reduces the risk of the development of some behavior problems, such as house soiling or intercat aggression.

Without pretraining, pets that are unaccustomed to confinement and separation from family members may vocalize, eliminate, and become destructive or anxious when separated from activities in the home. For most pets that do not have separation anxiety, training to be apart from an owner who is at home is fairly simple using the principles of desensitization. One should create a separate secure space (eg, a crate or a room with a baby gate or door) and then allow and encourage the pet to explore the space by putting treats or toys in the area. It may be useful to use a key phrase such as "go to your room" to place the behavior under verbal control. Once the pet is entering the space comfortably to look for rewards, the owner can start to acclimate the pet to being confined there for gradually increasing periods of time. One starts by confining the pet just long enough for it to finish a long-lasting treat. Then, over several sessions and over several days, one should increase the time the pet spends separated from the owner. Teaching a concurrent "settle" command is useful as well. If possible, cats should be confined in spaces that are large enough to hold a litter box as well as a comfortable resting area. If owners wish to teach a pet that has separation anxiety to be crated safely and comfortably, the process is similar but must proceed extremely slowly. A full behavior consultation is recommended in these cases to treat the separation anxiety and to assist the owners throughout the crate-training process (Fig. 1).

Sleeping Arrangements

With the exception of animals that are aggressive in beds or if disturbed while sleeping, there are no behavioral reasons to restrict pets from sleeping in bed with adult owners. Dogs and cats should have some practice sleeping apart from their owners, however, even if they typically share a bed. As mentioned earlier, this is good training for any pet, not just those who may experience an expanding family. Alternate sleeping arrangements may be on a dog bed or in a crate in the owner's bedroom or in a separate room of the house. If the pet has never spent the night apart from the owner, the owner should be prepared for the possibility of a few sleepless nights during the initial stages of the training process. The methods described earlier are used to make the pet

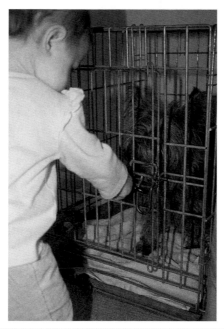

Fig. 1. Because small children often are interested in the pets in the house and quickly learn to open crates, this dog's owner has added an additional clip to secure the door to the kennel. (*Courtesy of* L. Bergman, VMD, Cayman Islands, BWI.)

comfortable with the chosen sleeping location during the day before trying to have it sleep there at night.

Feeding

The most trouble-free way to feed pets in a multipet household or in a household with children is meal feeding. In multipet households, meal feeding allows owners to control portions and diets for each individual animal and to determine accurately how much each pet consumes daily and reduces competition for food. In homes with children, meal feeding makes it easier to separate children from pets when they are eating. It is relatively easy to teach pets that have no history of food guarding to associate people approaching them while they eat with good things. Owners simply approach the pet while it is eating, say the pet's name or otherwise get its attention, and toss or drop a more delicious treat into the dish (eg, a piece of cheese or hot dog). After a few repetitions of receiving treats at a few different mealtimes, the pet should expect something good, and the owner can pet the animal and then give the treat. Although this training will not make a pet "childproof," it will reduce the likelihood that the pet will feel threatened by a person approaching while it eats. Not all dogs are responsive to this type of training. An easy alternative method to reduce feeding-related problems that should be used if dogs have any history of aggressively guarding food is to get the pets accustomed to eating alone behind some sort of sturdy barrier (eg, in a room that can be securely latched or closed in a crate) [2]. The food bowl should be picked up and put away after meal times in all situations. This location also should be used whenever the dog is given long-lasting treats, such as rawhides or bones. Food guarding is the most common reason for bites to children, according to one study, and 61% of dogs studied that had a history of biting children also had a history of aggressive resource guarding [3]. Even if dogs currently are not showing aggression toward their owners around food, it is common for this sort of aggression to resurface with the addition of new members of a household, whether children or other pets. Children should not be allowed to wander around the home with food while the dog is present, and in some cases it may be prudent to confine the dog securely while children are eating and perhaps when food is being prepared.

Handling

Pets should learn to tolerate, and possibly enjoy, handling all over their bodies. These steps can help prepare a pet for the sometimes less-than-gentle handling of a child but are not a guarantee that the animal will tolerate all forms of handling from the child. Veterinarians can demonstrate this handling during the physical examination while rewarding the pet with treats. If they notice that handling particular areas makes the pet seem tense or uncomfortable (eg, the animal pulls that body part away, licks its lips, or shows other signs of anxiety), they should demonstrate to the client how to desensitize and countercondition the pet to having these areas touched. As with all desensitization and counterconditioning, this process is done by introducing the stimulus at a level of intensity that causes no signs of anxiety and then rewarding the pet for being relaxed. The stimulus is increased gradually until it reaches a "real life" level. For example, if a cat does not like having its paws touched, the owner starts by gently stroking down the cat's legs, stopping at the first sign of any discomfort or ill-ease, such as ear flicking or tail twitching. While the stroking is taking place, the cat is given a treat it really enjoys, such as canned tuna fish. Over successive sessions, the owner's touch migrates down the cat's legs toward its feet. Once the owner is able to touch the cat's paws without its showing any anxiety, the touch is gradually built up from a brief stroke to actual holding. All the while, the cat is rewarded for remaining calm. At home, owners should handle their pets gently, over their entire bodies, as a matter of routine. As the pet becomes more comfortable with gentle handling, the owner gradually can begin to handle the pet in a slightly more clumsy and demanding manner, similar to that of a toddler, being careful not to hurt or scare the pet. The veterinarian should be sure that clients know that if the pet shows any aggression or other behaviors that make them nervous, they should stop these exercises altogether and arrange for a full behavioral consultation. When the animal already has a history of aggression during handling, a full behavior consultation is recommended before proceeding with this skill.

Politeness

A polite and well-mannered pet is one who has learned to have some self-control and to wait for permission before doing certain things, such as jumping onto furniture, exiting or entering the house or car, or going up and down stairs with owners. These behaviors can be taught easily through a policy of "nothing in life is free" [19] wherein the pet is given a simple command that it already knows well, such as "sit," before it is allowed to do any of the things that it wants to do [2,20]. Although this type of training most often is applied to dogs, variations can be used with cats. Depending on the activity level, size, and personality of the pet involved, owners may have to adjust how strict they are about enforcing their pet's politeness. The most important thing is consistency in enforcing the rules of the house with all pets and teaching the rules to children who are old enough to understand [21]. Once again, these behaviors are best taught through positive reinforcement [22].

ADDING CHILDREN TO THE HOME
General Considerations
Preparing pets for the arrival of a child, especially a baby or toddler, starts with preparing the house. Parents need to plan for how they will manage their pets, their children, and all of the paraphernalia that accompanies both human and animal family members. Expectant parents also need to plan not only for a stationary newborn but also for the active toddler that the baby soon will become. Any changes that directly affect the pet, such as moving litter boxes, feeding in a new location, or changing a dog-walking schedule should be made as far in advance of the arrival of the newcomer as possible. This approach allows the pet to get accustomed to these changes without the added challenges of adjusting to the child. If the pet is having a hard time adapting, the owners still have time to help the pet acclimate or to rethink how they will manage that aspect of their household routine before the family grows. Most importantly, if the pet does not adjust well to the change, the owners will not attribute all the problems to the arrival of a child.

For example, new parents may wait until their baby starts crawling to move the litter box to a babyproof location. If house soiling occurs, they blame it on jealousy or fear of the toddler, when the problem simply may be that the cat finds the new location unacceptable [2,23]. Encourage owners to keep litter boxes close to their current locations but in places that are usually childfree, such as home offices or master bedrooms/baths. Children can be kept out of these areas with baby gates (that cats can jump or that have small openings cut in them) or by propping doors open just wide enough for a cat to fit through [2].

Before children of any age arrive in the house, pet owners should begin implementing the following "skills for living with others," which are listed in order of importance: reward-based training, space and separation, nighttime sleeping, feeding, handling, and politeness. Expectant parents may want to practice some of these skills while holding realistic baby dolls. This technique can be especially useful for pets that are neophobic or very excitable [4].

INFANTS AND PETS

Dogs and cat should be introduced to all the paraphernalia that accompanies infants well in advance of the arrival of the infant. Dogs may need to learn to walk comfortably on leash next to strollers so that family walks can be a positive experience for the dog after the baby arrives [2,4]. Pets also should be acclimated to the noises associated with babies. The pet will be subjected to a crying infant, and a surprising amount of baby equipment produces high-pitched music and other sounds. Test noisy toys and devices in the presence of the pet, but not the baby, to see if the pet will be afraid of the sound or possibly even become aggressively aroused by it. If possible, the pet also should be exposed to the sounds of crying and laughing infants, either in person or via high-quality recordings [24]. If owners see their pets having problems, instructions for desensitizing the pet should be provided. Desensitization always starts by avoiding unnecessary exposure to the stimuli. Avoiding unnecessary exposure may require removing batteries from noisy toys to avoid turning them accidentally on or keeping the stroller in a closet. These items then can be taken out only for desensitization sessions during which the dog is rewarded for remaining calm when the item is present or being used.

Infants and Dogs

No dog should ever be left unattended with access to an infant or young child. Encourage clients to think about where they will be spending time during the day with their baby as well as their nighttime sleeping arrangements. There must be a means for physically separating dogs and children should a parent need to leave the room, even for only a moment to answer the telephone or use the bathroom. Sometimes it is easier to confine the baby in a crib or playpen than it is to confine the dog. If the dog is large enough to reach over the top of a playpen or strong enough to knock one over, however, the dog must not have access to the playpen or crib. Likewise, the dog should not have access to a baby in a swing, because several fatal dog maulings of unattended infants in swings have occurred [25]. Take every opportunity to remind expectant parents that no dog, no matter how good and trustworthy, ever should be left alone with an infant or small child. Similarly, if expectant parents are considering co-sleeping with their infant, they must plan for where their dog will sleep at night, especially if the dog has been sharing the owners' bed. It may be necessary to confine dogs physically at night so they do not get into family beds after the exhausted parents have fallen asleep.

New parents should be reminded that many baby toys and supplies, such as bottles, pacifiers, and teething rings are similar to dog toys. Once these items have been used or handled by a baby, they may have saliva or food residues on them that enhance their attractiveness to dogs. Recommendations for teaching dogs not to chew on things have been made elsewhere and typically involve providing alternatives, using taste aversion and/or booby traps, or keeping all items out of the dog's reach [20,26]. It can be very difficult to teach dogs to ignore these baby-related items, so avoidance is the best advice.

Because dogs may find dirty diapers attractive, one should advise dog owners to purchase a secure diaper pail and to test out the pail by knocking it over and trying to nudge it open themselves to avoid problems. If the dog will not be allowed in the nursery, this change should be implemented before the baby arrives.

Infants and Cats

Physically separating a cat from a baby that is not yet mobile usually is not as crucial as it is with a dog. Most cats, but not all, choose to avoid things that make them anxious [27]. Some cats, however, need to be taught to be comfortable being confined, either in a separate room of the house or in a large crate or cat condo. Cats that would benefit from this training are cats at either end of the fear–confidence spectrum: those that tend to react in a very fearful manner to stimuli or those that react in a more assertively aggressive manner. In the case of the very fearful cat, separation may be necessary, not for infant safety but because too much exposure to the infant may be extremely stressful for the cat. Although it is a myth that cats "snatch the breath" from babies, sleeping infants have been suffocated by cats that have sought out warm, soft resting places [28]. Expectant parents should not allow cats to sleep in cribs or strollers before the birth of the child with the assumption that the cat will not do so once the baby arrives. Crib tents and covers for strollers and playpens/portable cribs are available but are somewhat cumbersome. A good way to keep cats out of a baby's crib is to put a screen door across the nursery doorway. Doing so allows air to circulate, and caretakers still can hear the child, but pets cannot enter the room [2]. If this alternative is chosen, it should be implemented before the arrival of the child. Alternatively, cats can be confined at night, as recommended for dogs. Providing a "house of plenty" also will help by giving the cat sleeping or hiding options other than the baby's bed.

PET-TO-INFANT INTRODUCTIONS

After all the preparations for the arrival of a new infant have been explained to pet owners, the next step is to discuss the actual homecoming and introduction of the infant. If possible, new parents should bring home clothes or blankets with the baby's scent before the baby comes home. The owners should let the pets familiarize themselves with the baby's scent and give the pets treats for calmly sniffing these items [4]. It is common for pets to show the flehmen response when sniffing newborns; this behavior usually is not a cause for concern. When the baby first arrives home, it is best that pets not be given free access to the owners or baby. If a pet has not spent significant time with its owners for several days, the new parents should spend some time reuniting with the pet apart from the baby before making the introduction. In particular, a new mother should enter the house empty-handed to avoid problems with dogs trying to jump up in greeting. Once the pets are calm and the baby is either sleeping calmly or awake but not crying, the first introduction to the child can take place. Dogs should be on leash with a responsible adult controlling access to the infant. For some excitable dogs, a head collar will allow for additional calming and control. This device should be introduced well in advance of the baby's arrival. How slowly to proceed with the introduction depends on the dog's previous history with children and its general reaction to new things. For most dogs it is adequate to keep the dog on leash and give it treats for calmly sniffing the baby. As long as the pet is interested, but not overly excited, it can be allowed to continue to sniff the baby. If the pet seems to be getting too excited or fearful, its attention should be directed gently to another activity, such as reward-based training or playing with a toy. If the pet's attention cannot be redirected easily, or if any signs of aggression are seen, it should be led calmly and quietly away from the baby without any type of punishment [2,4,29]. It is equally important that the owners do not force the pets to interact with the baby (eg, picking up a cat and holding it next to the infant). The pet should be allowed to investigate the newcomer gently on its own terms (Fig. 2) [2].

For dogs that are more fearful or excitable, introductions may be smoother if a distance is maintained between the dog and the baby. The owners should reward the dog for remaining calm and performing basic commands while the distance between dog and baby is gradually decreased. With dogs that are likely to have difficulty remaining calm in this setting, the initial introduction(s) can be made over the course of several days during family walks [2,4].

Even if the initial introduction has gone well, new parents should strengthen their pet's positive associations with the baby over the first few weeks. They can do so by giving the pets special treats or attention when the baby is near, especially if the baby is crying, and by taking dogs on family walks with the baby in a stroller or carrier. A common pitfall is to ignore the pet when the baby is awake and shower the pet with attention when the baby is sleeping. The baby being present and, especially, being awake should signal to the dog that good things, such as getting treats, walks, and social interaction, will happen. The absence of the baby should mean that nothing special will

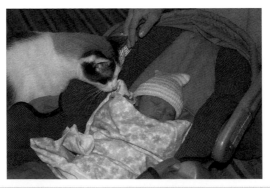

Fig. 2. After greeting her pets while her newborn sleeps, this mother supervises her cat's first introduction to the baby. (*Courtesy of* J. Capaldo, DVM, San Diego, CA.)

happen but not that the dog is totally ignored. For example, if the owners and dog are used to snuggling on the couch in the evenings, they should continue to do this after the baby is in bed to maintain some degree of their familiar routine. For an anxious animal this level of disruption of the pet's normal interactions with the owners may be a source of extra stress and anxiety added to the new addition to the family. Instead, the pet should receive some attention and affection even when the baby is not present, with very special treats and attention reserved for times that the baby is near. Owners also can take advantage of times when the baby is sleeping to do things with the dog that may be done best without involving small children. These activities may be things that the dog enjoys, like some types of play that may result in rambunctious behavior, which could knock over a small child. This also is a good time for owners to do things, like grooming, that the dog may not enjoy. This way, the dog will not associate these experiences with the baby, and the child will not try to mimic the parents.

TODDLERS, OLDER CHILDREN, AND PETS

Dogs and cats actually are more likely to have problems with toddlers and older children than with infants [30]. Fortunately, in most homes, the parents have a chance to prepare for the maturing child to become more mobile and independent. This oportunity may not exist in blended families. In these circumstances, the pets should be introduced to the children through meetings at neutral locations or during short, supervised visits before the children and pets begin living together. The dog should be kept on leash and allowed to approach the child, who should be seated, provided the dog and child are calm. The dog's calmness can be reinforced through simple commands. Head collars may allow additional calming and control in some dogs. Older children should be instructed to maintain a nonthreatening body posture (eg, sitting down, staying still) and to refrain from yelling or grabbing at the dog. The child should toss or hand treats to the dog, depending on how comfortable each seems with the other. Playing fetch is another good initial interaction for children and dogs if the dog will give up the object willingly [4,20]. A similar approach can be used with cats, although these introductions are made best in a location where the cat feels comfortable, rather than moving to a neutral territory. Playtime with a cat also can be used to facilitate introductions.

Preparing pets to live with toddlers and older children is similar to the steps described for infants, with one notable difference. As the children involved get older, they will be more involved in learning to interact appropriately with their pets. It is never too early for parents to start teaching their children how to behave safely and appropriately around dogs and cats. Parents, however, should be aware that young children cannot be relied on to keep interactions with animals safe. After food guarding, the second most common situations in which children under the age of 6 years were bitten by familiar dogs involved activities like falling onto or stepping on dogs or pulling their fur [3]. Although some of these situations, like falling on a dog, are caused by the child's stage of physical development, others, like pulling fur, may be caused by a young child's inability to understand how to be gentle. Children under the age of 4 years are particularly inept at interpreting dog behavior, especially in interpreting friendly and fearful behaviors [31]. For older children, the most common situations resulting in bites involved activities typically considered benign, such as petting, hugging, and kissing dogs [3]. Parents may be able to mitigate some of these problems by educating their children about how to be safe with animals. One promising resource for parents of children aged 3 to 6 years is The Blue Dog Project, an interactive dog bite prevention CD [32]. The recommendation for separating unsupervised pets and children is the same as for infants. Depending on the behavior of the pet and the maturity level of the child, this separation may need to continue until the child is approaching preteen years.

In addition to separating dogs from children during the dogs' mealtimes, dog-owning parents should teach their children that their meals and snacks are eaten while sitting down at a table. Clients may be more likely to comply with this recommendation if they are reminded that it follows pediatricians' guidelines to prevent choking, as well as denying the dogs easy access to the children's food (Fig. 3) [33].

PROBLEMS AND PITFALLS

The greatest concern that most pet owners have about adding children to a household with existing pets is that the pets will harm the children. This fear often is the factor driving expectant parents to seek veterinary advice.

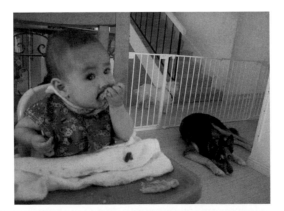

Fig. 3. This picture shows that the dogs in this house are separated from the feeding child based on their ability to remain calm and not bother the baby, not based on their size. (*Courtesy of* J. Capaldo, DVM, San Diego, CA.)

Although infants can be injured by pets, with horrific consequences [25,28,30], they actually are at less risk than children between the ages of 1 to 9 years [3,30]. Most aggression has an anxiety component, and fear-based aggression is the most likely diagnosis for dogs that bite children [3]. Owners often assume the aggression is caused by dominance, but this cause is unlikely when a small child is involved. (There may be competition for space with crawling children, however, because a crawling child occupies the same space as the dog, something to which the pet may not be accustomed.) A careful history usually reveals other behaviors as well as body language that are consistent with fear [3,29]. As noted earlier, these dogs may have a history of other anxieties, a lack of early socialization to children, or a prior history of aggression to children [3,4,34]. Treating pets that are fearful and/or aggressive to children involves a judicious combination of management (avoidance) and desensitization. Animals with a past or present history of aggression to children should have a full behavior consultation that goes beyond the general advice given to most pet owners.

Predatory behavior may be involved in some attacks on infants and very young children [2,25,29]. In these situations, the pet typically does not show the threat behaviors (eg, growling, baring teeth) or anxious behaviors (eg, pinning ears back, lowered [but not crouching like an animal that is about to pounce] body posture, or holding the tail down) that may accompany other forms of aggression. These animals are focused on the infant and may become highly aroused simply by hearing the infant. They may attempt to seek out the baby, and their arousal may be enhanced by movement (eg, in a swing or stroller) or by sounds from toys [25]. These animals are very dangerous because they do not appear to perceive the infant as a person but simply as a prey item. Because this behavior can be thought of as a normal behavior directed at an abnormal target, predatory aggression can be very hard to change through behavior modification [35]. The best way to keep children safe from these pets is through strict separation. In some cases, it may be necessary to remove the pet from the household. If the pet has a history of being nonaggressive toward older children, the pet can be returned to the home when the child has reached an age at which he or she is no longer viewed as prey. Although predatory aggression may be anticipated based on the pet's behavior toward other animals, especially prey species, this behavior is not a reliable indicator and should not be used to make absolute recommendations about re-homing or euthanasia. One author (LB) has personal experience with a terrier that is an accomplished hunter but viewed her newborn daughter as a person and displayed behaviors toward the baby that it shows only toward people.

For dogs that show fearful behaviors toward infants, it sometimes is recommended that owners completely ignore their dog when the baby is not present, to make the association of good things happening when the baby is near more potent [29]. This technique is best reserved for use in a comprehensive behavioral treatment plan, following a full behavior consultation, in which its effects and side effects can be monitored. As noted earlier, as general advice for acclimating most pets, this approach probably is too extreme and places a heavy burden on the new parents.

PET-TO-PET INTRODUCTIONS
General Considerations

Predicting how interactions will proceed when adding a new pet to an existing household may be difficult, but veterinarians can recommend steps to decrease the risk of problems and increase the chance of a successful outcome. Although introductions between resident and newly adopted dogs have not been researched, adding a new dog to the household often is cited as a cause of aggression between two household dogs [36]. Dog-to-dog introductions have been studied in dog parks, and results indicate that very few first meetings on neutral territory result in fights [37,38]. One study assessed introductions of a newly adopted shelter cat to a household in which one or more cats already resided [39]. Fifty percent of these households reported initial aggression (scratching and biting), and aggression was more likely to continue for some time if the first introduction was unfriendly. So, if the initial meeting between two pets can be controlled and set up to succeed, the final integration of the new pet into the household may be successful also.

The safety of the pets and people involved and control of the introductions should be the most important topics when discussing new introductions with clients. All dogs should be comfortable on leash and have a few basic commands that were taught with positive reinforcement [22]. These skills can be advantageous for cat introductions also, and all cats should be comfortable being confined in a separate room.

For feline introductions, it is best to keep cats safely separated initially so the resident cat can become familiar with the new sounds and odors of the newcomer [5]. Allowing auditory and olfactory information to be transmitted without the additional stimulus of seeing the other cat may help to make the introduction more successful. This exposure can be accomplished by keeping cats in separate rooms and rotating rooms daily or by transferring scent by sequentially petting each cat with the same cloth [40]. Rotating rooms also allows newcomers to become comfortable with their new home without the added challenge of adjusting to other animals. This approach is especially important for cats that tend to be neophobic. Keeping all cats indoors may decrease the risk of problems, because fighting is more likely to occur [39] in response new odors or to re-establish status [41] after a cat returns from outside.

One should advise clients that once cats are comfortable with access to each other's space, smells, and sounds, they may be fed on separate sides of the door to the room the newcomer is occupying. Encouraging a pleasurable activity in the presence of the other cat classically conditions the cats to enjoy each other's company. Once cats are comfortable with this feeding arrangement, they can be given visual but not physical access to each other while eating by blocking the door so it stays ajar or by stacking baby gates or putting a screen door in the doorway. Another option is to put the cats in carriers for feeding and gradually move them closer to each other with each meal. For this approach to be successful, the cats must show nonaggressive and nonfearful body language continually throughout the introductions. If the introduction is gradual enough for the cats, the owner will observe only good behavior from both of them. The time it takes for this to occur is up to the pets, not the owners. The owners can facilitate it, but they cannot force the issue; otherwise they probably will cause more problems.

Excitement has been found to be the most common trigger for fighting between household dogs, followed by food and toys [42]. These stimuli should be avoided during an initial meeting [36]. Clients should maintain an upbeat and jolly attitude without overly exciting the dogs [43]. Introductions can be made in a park or during a long walk near the new dog, preferably on leash for safety and control. For dogs that exhibit aggression toward other dogs when on leash but not off leash, this recommendation may have to be modified. Owners should praise normal, calm greeting behaviors and read the dogs' body language to assess the situation, looking for tails and ears that are in neutral to slightly drooped (but not tucked) positions, tail wagging and any signs of play, and submissive but not fearful behavior. If the dogs are getting along, they can be taken into the house. Once in the house, asking dogs to perform behaviors they know, such as sit or down, for minute pieces of treats conditions them to enjoy being in each other's company.

Because crowding is a primary environmental factor that may increase aggression, the pets should be given as much room as possible [6]. Indoor cats have been shown to section off the interior of the house and use specific rooms as their territory or to timeshare common areas [44,45]. A space as small as little as 10 square meters per cat in the house can result in no fighting and little aggression [44], depending on the temperament of the individual cats. Maintaining a house of plenty, as discussed earlier, can help decrease tension [46]. Dogs typically prefer to be within 23 inches of each other [47], but if they meet in a hallway or one is cornered in some way, aggression may be used to increase the distance between them.

Even if the initial meeting between two pets is uneventful, owners should not assume that the animals now are great friends and can be left alone together. The best advice is to keep unsupervised pets safely and securely separated with their own beds or resting spots, food and water dishes, and toys. The first few times they are together they should be kept safe and controlled on loose leashes; if problems arise, the clients should move the animals calmly away from each other. Reading the pets' body language is essential to determine when to stop an interaction, before aggression or fear occurs. Good behavior in the presence of the other pet should be rewarded with something the pet enjoys, such as calm praise, petting, or a small treat. Verbal or physical punishment of pets for undesirable behavior toward each other only increases tension and anxiety and is not recommended.

The veterinarian should help clients make an informed decision on pet selection and use common sense. A dog or cat that has a history of aggression to other dogs, cats, or other pet species may not be the best choice of a pet to add to an existing household (see the article by Duxbury and Marder elsewhere in this issue). If introducing more than one pet to another, clients should introduce them in pairs first, as outlined earlier, to avoid overwhelming the animals.

Problems that May Occur

One reason that problems occur during new pet introductions is lack of patience on the part of the owners. Clients want their pets to get along and want it happen fast. In one study of cat introductions, 44% of people put the cats together immediately [39]. When cats were housed singly in quarantine situations, it took 5 weeks for the cats to adapt to the new environment [48]. It may be even more stressful and take more time for cats to adjust when introduced to a household that is ever changing and has other pets.

Other reasons for problems relate to the temperament, genetics, and social experiences of the animals involved [41,49]. If newcomers are obtained from shelters or rescue organizations, their previous behaviors and experience may be unknown. In most cases temperament tests do not predict future behaviors accurately [50] (see the article by Duxbury and Marder elsewhere in this issue), and even if they did, relationships between animals are never static. For this reason, owners need to monitor the relationship continually and reward good behaviors intermittently.

Aggression is the most obvious and risky problem that may develop when introducing new pets to an existing household. The motivation for aggression may be territorial, fear, redirected aggression, status, food-related aggression, or predation. Dogs and cats are territorial species by nature, and their territory is the space that is defended actively from intrusion. Dogs show more aggression as the intruder moves closer to the center of their territory [51]. Cats show more aggression when there is an influx of new cats or a high density of cats and when they are unable to leave the area [52].

Dogs that are territorial in the house or the yard may redirect aggression onto each other if thwarted from interacting with the target of their aggression. Redirected aggression can occur between cats during an initial meeting; unusual noises and odors are some of the common triggers involved [5,53]. Cats have long memories for the victims towards which they redirect aggression, so the problem usually escalates after an initial episode if the cats remain together [5].

The resident cat may react to the newcomer with fear, which may lead to defensive aggression [39,54]. If the frightened cat cannot escape when an approaching animal reaches the cat's critical distance, defensive aggression may occur until escape is possible [5]. Social encounters between dogs may elicit fear [51], which again may result in aggression if a dog is cornered.

Status aggression should be considered when a cat uses aggression to control a situation. If the resident cat is assertive and confident in nature, such control may be the motivation for aggression towards the newly added cat [41]. The social status among dogs may change when a new dog is added to the household, and aggression may result involving any or all of the dogs [36].

Possession- or food-related aggression may be seen during initial introductions of dogs if the owners have not removed all these items. Even if the resident dog has never shown aggression toward people in regards to food or possessions, this aggression may manifest when a resource is threatened by a conspecific [55]. Cats rarely fight over food, instead adopting a first-come/first-served attitude [5]. For cats that may fight over food, a house of plenty will decrease the risk of this occurring.

Dogs may act in a predatory fashion toward cats, and dog and cats may predate other small pets [55]. This behavior is a normal instinct but can be highly dangerous when directed toward other pets. If pets have been socialized to prey species from an early age, the risk may be lessened but not eliminated. Once a cat starts hunting, the behavior can be very difficult to prevent [5].

Fear and anxiety caused by the new living situation can cause problems other than aggression. House soiling may occur because of unfamiliarity with the new toileting area or because interactions between pets inhibit a pet's access to the toileting area. Cats may have additional issues such as too few litter boxes or uncleanliness. Urine marking may occur and may be related to territorial issues and/or anxiety in dogs [56] and cats [57]. (see the article by Levine elsewhere in this issue). Some animals may show a decrease in appetite after the addition of a new pet because of emotional stress [58], and a subordinate dog may refuse to eat in the presence of more confident dogs [35]. Anxiety may be manifested as social withdrawal or escape behaviors. If clients become impatient and try to force an animal into interacting, this enforced interaction also may lead to fear-related aggression. Anxiety in animals also can manifest as self-directed or compulsive behaviors such as tail chasing in dogs [59]. If these behavioral manifestations of stress and anxiety are the presenting complaints, the veterinarian needs to question the client about the family situation of the pets.

TREATMENT OF PROBLEMS

The treatment for the individual problem behaviors differs depending on the diagnosis made. Determining the motivation behind the problem behavior requires a thorough behavioral history. For issues between a pet and children, the clients must to be questioned about the pet's previous experiences with children, how the children interact with and feel about the pet, and how the parents are managing the pet and the children. For problems between pets, the information needed includes how the clients interact with each of the pets, whether they favor one pet over the other, and if tension exists between the clients about acquisition of the new pet or on how to proceed with treatment. Once a diagnosis is made, treatment plans can be found in other sources [29,55,60,61].

It always is good advice to keep children and pets safely separated from each other until a thorough work-up can be performed and a customized treatment plan can be devised for that particular household. Separation helps in many situations because it decreases everyone's tension and anxiety, which may be the underlying cause of the problem behavior. Separation does not address or treat the problem, so unless the clients want the children and/or pets to live in the same house but apart, behavioral treatment is needed. If adjunctive therapies such as pheromones and aromatherapy were not used during the initial introduction, they may be recommended if problems arise.

If aggression is the primary concern, clients can prepare for behavioral therapy by accustoming the dogs involved to wearing head collars and basket muzzles, using positive reinforcement. Aggressive cats should be accustomed to body harnesses and cat carriers, also using positive reinforcement. Referral to a veterinary behaviorist is warranted because of the high risk of injury involved.

During a full behavior consultation, owners must be given an assessment of the risks to their children, to visiting children [34,62], and to other pets. Discussions of how to manage the household safely to avoid injuries, what would be involved in behavior modification, the possible use of medications and their side effects, as well as a prognosis must take place. This information allows the owners to make an informed decision about whether to attempt to manage the situation and treat the pet or to remove the pet from the household. Realistic expectations of the outcome of treatment for any behavioral problem must be addressed, because some animals may be able to live together harmoniously and yet not get along to the client's satisfaction. Owners also should be given a realistic appraisal of the likelihood of re-homing the particular pet, given what is known about the pet's behavior. In some circumstances, re-homing may not be a realistic option, and euthanasia must be discussed [2].

Further Readings
Available at: http://www.vetmedpub.com/vetmed/data/articlestandard/vetmed/422006/379302/article.pdf.
Available at: http://www.dogsandkids.ca/.
Available at: http://www.thebluedog.org.

References
[1] Bergman L, Hart BL, Bain MJ, et al. Evaluation of urine marking by cats as a model for understanding veterinary diagnostic and treatment approaches and client attitudes. J Am Vet Med Assoc 2002;221(6):1282–6.

[2] Bergman L. Ensuring a behaviorally healthy pet-child relationship. Vet Med 2006;101(23):670–80.

[3] Reisner I, Shofer F, Nance M. Behavioral assessment of child-directed canine aggression. Inj Prev 2007;23:348–51.

[4] Lindsay S. Impulsive, extrafamilial, and intraspecific aggression. In: Handbook of applied dog behavior and training: procedures and protocols, vol. 3. Ames (IA): Blackwell Publishing; 2005. p. 433–555.

[5] Beaver BV. Feline social behavior. In: Feline behavior: a guide for veterinarians. 2nd edition. St Louis (MO): Saunders; 2003. p. 127–63.

[6] Houpt KA. Aggression and social structure. In: Domestic animal behavior for veterinarians and animal scientists. 2nd edition. Ames (IA): Iowa State Univ Press; 1991. p. 34–74.

[7] Shepard K. Development of behaviour, social behaviour and communication in dogs. In: Horwitz D, Mills D, Heath S, editors. BSAVA manual of canine and feline behavioural medicine. Quedgeley, Gloucester (UK): British Small Animal Veterinary Association; 2002. p. 23–23.

[8] Heath S. Feline aggression. In: Horowitz D, Mills D, Heath S, editors. BSAVA manual of canine and feline behavioural medicine. Quedgeley, Gloucester (UK): British Small Animal Veterinary Association; 2002. p. 216–28.

[9] Doggone crazy. Available at: www.doggonecrazy.ca.

[10] Pageat P, Gaultier E. Current research in canine and feline pheromones In: Vet Clin North Am 2003;33:187–211.

[11] Pageat P, Tessier Y. Usefulness of the F3 synthetic pheromone Feliway in preventing behavior problems in cats during holidays. Presented of the International Conference on Veterinary Behavioural Medicine. Birmingham, United Kingdom, April 1–2, 1997.

[12] Schwartz S. Western psychoactive herbs. In: Psychoactive herbs in veterinary behavior medicine. Ames (IA): Blackwell Publishing, Ltd; 2005. p. 3–93.

[13] Clark G, Boyer W. The effects of dog obedience training and behavioral counseling upon human-canine relationship. Appl Anim Behav Sci 1993;37:147–59.

[14] Raupp C. Treasuring, trashing or terrorizing: adult outcomes of childhood socialization about companion animals. Soc Anim 1999;23(2):121–59.

[15] Ascoine FR, Webber CW. Children's attitudes about the humane treatment of animals and empathy: one-year follow up of a school-based intervention. Anthrozoos 1995;23(4): 190–4.

[16] Schalke E, Stichnoth J, Ott S, et al. Clinical signs caused by the use of electric training collars on dogs in everyday life situations. Appl Anim Behav Sci 2007;105:369–80.

[17] Reisner I. An overview of aggression. In: Horwitz D, Mills D, Heath S, editors, BSAVA manual of canine and feline behavioural medicine. vol 1. Quedgeley, Gloucester (UK): British Small Animal Veterinary Association; 2002. p. 181–94.

[18] American Veterinary Society of Animal Behavior Web site. Available at: http://www. avsabonline.org/avsabonline/images/stories/avsab%20punishguidelines.pdf.

[19] Voith V, Borchelt PL. Diagnosis and treatment of dominance aggression in dogs. Vet Clin North Am Small Anim Pract 1982;12:655–63.

[20] Hetts S. Pet behavior protocols: what to say, what to do, when to refer. Lakewood (CO): AAHA Press; 1999.

[21] Eskeland GE, Tillung RH, Bakken M. The importance of consistency in the training of dogs. The effect of punishment, rewards, control and attitude on obedience and problem behaviours in dogs. In: Proceedings of the International Veterinary Behaviour Meeting. Riccione (Italy): Fandazione Iniziative Zooprofilattiche e Zootecniche; 2007. p. 179–180.

[22] Hiby EF, Rooney NJ, Bradshaw JWS. Dog training methods; their use, effectiveness and interaction with behaviour and welfare. Anim Welf 2004;23:63–9.

[23] Olm DD, Houpt KA. Feline house-soiling problems. Appl Anim Behav Sci 1988;20: 335–45.

[24] Sound therapy 4 pets Sounds Soothing CD. Available at: http://www.soundtherapy4pets. com/.

[25] Chu AY, Ripple MG, Allan CH, et al. Fatal dog maulings associated with infant swings. J Forensic Sci 2006;51(2):403–6.

[26] Lindell E. Control problems in dogs. In: Horwitz D, Mills D, Heath S, editors. BSAVA manual of canine and feline behavioural medicine. Quedgeley, Gloucester (UK): British Small Animal Veterinary Association; 2002. p. 69–79.

[27] Casey R. Fear and stress. In: Horwitz D, Mills D, Heath S, editors. BSAVA manual of canine and feline behavioural medicine. Quedgeley, Gloucester (UK): British Small Animal Veterinary Association; 2002. p. 144–53.

[28] Kearney MS, Dahl LB, Stalsberg H. Can a cat smother and kill a baby? Br Med J 1982;285: 777.

[29] Hart BL, Hart LA, Bain MJ. Canine and feline behavior therapy. 2nd edition. Ames (IA): Blackwell Publishing; 2006. p. 103–28.

[30] Overall KL, Love M. Dog bites to humans—demography, epidemiology, injury, and risk. J Am Vet Med Assoc 2001;218(23):1923–34.

[31] Lakestani NN, Donaldson M, Verga M, et al. Keeping children safe: how reliable are children at interpreting dog behavior? Presented at the 40th International Congress of the International Society for Applied Ethology. Bristol, United Kingdom, August 23–23, 2006.

[32] Meints K, De Keuster T. Test yourself—a first assessment of the dog bite prevention project "Blue Dog." Available at: http://www.vin.com/members/proceedings/proceedings.plx?CID=WSAVA2006&PID=16096&0=Generic.

[33] American Academy of Pediatrics. Patenting corner Q&A: choking prevention. Available at: http://www.aap.org/publiced/BR_Choking.htm.

[34] Mertens P. Canine aggression. In: Horwitz D, Mill D, Heath S, editors. BSAVA manual of canine and feline behavioural medicine. Quedgeley, Gloucester (UK): British Small Animal Veterinary Association; 2002. p. 195–215.

[35] Bowen J. Miscellaneous behavior problems. In: Horwitz DF, Mill DS, Heath S, editors. BSAVA manual of canine and feline behavioural medicine. Gloucester (UK): British Small Animal Veterinary Association; 2002. p. 119–27.

[36] Horwitz DF, Neilson JC. Aggression/canine: interdog/familiar dogs. In: Blackwell's five-minute veterinary consult: canine and feline behavior. Ames (IA): Blackwell Publishing; 2007. p. 63–70.

[37] Bradshaw JWS, Lee A. Dyadic interactions between domestic dogs. Anthrozoos 1993; 5(4):245–53.

[38] Shyan MR, Fortune KA, King C. Bark parks—a study on interdog aggression in a limited control environment. J Appl Anim Welfare Sci 2003;6(1):25–32.

[39] Levine ES, Perry P, Scarlett J, et al. Intercat aggression in households following the introduction of a new cat. Appl Anim Behav Sci 2005;90:325–36.

[40] Horwitz DF, Neilson JC. Appendix D handouts. In: Blackwell's five-minute veterinary consult: canine and feline behavior. Ames (IA): Blackwell Publishing; 2007. p. 548–80.

[41] Landsberg G, Hunthausen W, Ackerman L. Feline aggression. In: Handbook of behavior problems of the dog and cat. 2nd edition. Edinburg (TX): Elsevier Saunders; 2003. p. 427–53.

[42] Sherman C. Characteristics, treatment, and outcome of 99 cases of aggression between dogs. Appl Anim Behav Sci 1996;47(1/2):91–108.

[43] Campbell WE. Aggressive behavior. In: Behavior problems in dogs. Santa Barbara (CA): American Veterinary Publications; 1975. p. 179–232.

[44] Bernstein PL, Strack M. A game of cat and house: spatial patterns and behavior of 23 domestic cats (Felis catus) in the home. Anthrozoos 1996;23(1):25–39.

[45] Bernstein P, Strack M. Home ranges, favored spots, time-sharing patterns, and tail usage by 14 cats in the home. Animal Behavior Consultants Newsletter 1993;10(3):1–3.

[46] Neilson J. Thinking outside the box: feline elimination. J Feline Med Surg 2004;6(1):5–23.

[47] Fuller JL, Fox MW. The behaviour of dogs. In: Hafez ESE, editor. The behaviour of domestic animals. 2nd edition. Baltimore (MD): Williams and Wilkins Co; 1969. p. 433–81.

[48] Rochlitz I, Podberscek AL, Broom DM. Welfare of cats in a quarantine cattery. Vet Rec 1998;143(2):35–9.

[49] Svartberg K. Breed-typical behaviour in dogs—historical remnants or recent constructs? Appl Anim Behav Sci 2005;96:293–313.

[50] Jones AC, Gosling SD. Temperament and personality in dogs (Canis familiaris): a review and evaluation of past research. Appl Anim Behav Sci 2005;95:1–53.

[51] Beaver BV. Canine social behavior. In: Canine behavior: a guide for veterinarians. Philadelphia: W.B.Saunders; 1999. p. 137–99.

[52] Wolski TR. Social behavior of the cat. Vet Clin North Am Small Anim Pract 1982;23(4): 693–706.

[53] Amat M, Manteca X, Fatjo J. Animal behavior case of the month. J Am Vet Med Assoc 2007;231(5):710–2.
[54] Borchelt PL, Voith VL. Diagnosis and treatment of aggression problems in cats. Vet Clin North Am Small Anim Pract 1982;23(4):665–71.
[55] Overall KL. Clinical behavioral medicine for small animals. St. Louis (MO): Mosby-Year Book, Inc.; 1997.
[56] Beaver BV. Canine eliminative behavior. In: Canine behavior: a guide for veterinarians. Philadelphia: W.B.Saunders; 1999. p. 267–87.
[57] Beaver BV. Feline eliminative behavior. In: Feline behavior: a guide for veterinarians. St Louis (MO): Saunders; 2003. p. 247–73.
[58] Beaver BV. Feline ingestive behavior. In: Feline behavior: a guide for veterinarians. St Louis (MO): Saunders; 2003. p. 212–46.
[59] Landsberg G, Hunthausen W, Ackerman L. Stereotypic and compulsive disorders. In: Handbook of behavior problems of the dog and cat. 2nd edition. Edinburgh (TX): Elsevier Saunders; 2003. p. 195–225.
[60] Landsberg G, Hunthausen W, Ackerman L. Handbook of behavior problems of the dog and cat. 2nd edition. Edinburgh (TX): Elsevier Saunders; 2003.
[61] Horwitz DF, Neilson JC. Blackwell's five-minute veterinary consult: canine and feline behavior. 1st edition. Ames (IA): Blackwell publishing; 2007.
[62] Lindsay SR. Handbook of applied dog behavior and training. vol 2. 1st edition. Ames (IA): Iowa State University Press; 2001.

Vet Clin Small Anim 38 (2008) 1065–1079

VETERINARY CLINICS
SMALL ANIMAL PRACTICE

Feline Fear and Anxiety

Emily D. Levine, DVM, MRCVS

Animal Emergency and Referral Associates, 1237 Bloomfield Avenue, Fairfield, NJ 07004, USA

M any behavioral problems in cats stem from underlying anxiety or fears. Therefore, an understanding of how emotions contribute to, cause, and exacerbate behavior problems is crucial in implementing appropriate treatment plans. In addition, a basic understanding of how emotions affect the physiologic stress response is paramount, because this has serious implications in the cat's overall mental and physical well-being and influences the decision to use psychoactive medications. The purpose of this article is, first, to review the relation between stress and emotions and pertinent physiology; second, to identify some common feline behavioral problems seen as a result of underlying fear and anxiety; and third, to outline treatment principles for those problems.

EMOTIONS AND STRESS

Theories by psychologists James and Carl Lange propose that the physiologic stress responses (eg, increased heart rate, respiratory rate) occur first and that these responses lead to the feelings of fear and anxiety. Others have criticized this theory and propose that it is the emotion that precedes and causes the physiologic stress response, which serves as the secondary assisting mechanism enabling the animal's ability to react or cope with the emotion (eg, fear, anxiety) [1]. Many of those in the field of animal behavior, animal cognition, and animal welfare are likely to subscribe to the second theory.

As veterinarians, we are traditionally trained to be concerned with the physiologic consequences of stress, and not necessarily with the emotional states that are likely to be initiating those physiologic consequences. By acknowledging the importance of emotions in the role of behavior, stress, and disease, we may be more successful in treating diseases (eg, feline lower urinary tract disease [FLUTD]) known to be caused or exacerbated by stress [2–4] and, of course, behavior problems for which underlying fear or anxiety is an important component (eg, intercat aggression, spraying). To begin to understand the relation between stress and emotions, consistent working definitions must be given.

Stress is currently a widely used term for describing complex and not well-understood cognitive, emotional, and somatic responses to various stimuli,

E-mail address: dremilylevine@hotmail.com

0195-5616/08/$ – see front matter
doi:10.1016/j.cvsm.2008.04.010

some pleasant stimuli, and some aversive stimuli [1]. Although the term *stress* is broad and nonspecific, most agree that a basic tenet of stress is that its goal is to maintain physiologic and psychologic homeostasis [1]. The stress response is seen with pleasurable and aversive situations and activities; thus, physiologic stress does not always indicate an unpleasant situation but rather a change from the normal homeostatic state of the animals. Stress is a physiologic response activated by emotions (eg, fear, anxiety) to assist the animal in coping with the emotion and should be considered a normal healthy response in the short term.

For the purposes of this article, distress is defined as behavioral or physiologic responses that have deleterious effects on an animal's welfare [5]. Although stress is an important and necessary part of everyday life, when the coping response is unable to eliminate the source of fear or anxiety, the coping response can be harmful when activated for a long period and is now called distress.

Fear is an emotion that induces an adaptive response ("stress response") enabling an animal to avoid situations and activities that could be dangerous [6]. The emotional response is initiated when an animal perceives a threatening stimulus and induces a primary behavioral response that protects it from the perceived threatening stimulus, which is clearly identifiable. Fear is normal and appropriate in certain situations. If the animal is unable to remove itself from the fearful situation or the attempt to get away from the fearful stimuli fails, fear may lead to chronic states of anxiety (which may present as aggression).

Anxiety is an emotional response to an unidentifiable stimulus or may result from the inability to escape or control situations that elicit an initial fear response [7]. The latter comment, in the author's opinion, is a key factor in intercat aggression and spraying cases, because household cats are often unable to control factors in their environment or behave in ways that eliminate sources of fear; therefore, they are living in an ongoing anxious state.

PATHOPHYSIOLOGY: ANXIETY, FEAR, STRESS

The stress response and the emotions of fear and anxiety involve similar central nervous system (CNS) structures—the thalamic tracts, amygdala, and hypothalamus, which helps to prepare the animal by increasing cortical arousal and alertness and preparing the body for rapid defense [8]. Despite shared neuroanatomic pathways, fear and stress are not the same thing. Studies have demonstrated that sympathetic activation does not alone produce feelings of fear [9,10]. When an animal perceives a stimulus as aversive or frightening, a part of the brain essential to fear responses, the amygdala, is triggered. Stimulation of the amygdala activates the hypothalamic-pituitary-adrenal (HPA) axis [11]. Although the stress response in the short term is healthy, when the response is prolonged, physical and emotional pathologic conditions ensue. Interestingly, studies have shown that psychologic factors can be more potent factors in stimulating the HPA axis than physical factors [12]. It is this concept that makes understanding animal behavior and their "merkwelt" (ie, perceptual world) so important in treating behavioral problems successfully and humanely.

Historically, the stress response has been perceived as a single invariant stress response; however, more recently, it is being perceived as a diverse array of different patterns of physiologic changes when an animal encounters different aversive stimuli [13–15]. The latter perception of the stress response helps to illuminate the importance of addressing each feline patient as an individual when devising treatment plans for behavioral issues, because each cat is likely to react or respond to stress in different ways. Despite the individual differences in the stress response, there are some common pathways that are stimulated when an animal feels anxious, fearful, or stressed. Two important systems that respond are the sympathoadrenal (SA) response and the HPA response. These responses serve to enhance and assist the body to deal with the emotion that stimulated them. Certainly the first system to be engaged is that of the SA system to release epinephrine and norepinephrine from the adrenal gland and subcortical areas of the brain [16]. These hormones are responsible for the classic fight, flight, or freeze response and prepare and enable the animal to respond physiologically. The heart rate increases, cardiac output is greater, the respiration rate increases, and there is peripheral vasoconstriction to organ systems not needed in immediately threatening situations (eg, gastrointestinal system). Epinephrine stimulates glycolysis, gluconeogenesis, and lipolysis, which helps to keep a ready source of energy for sustained fleeing or fighting. With the physiologic changes primed, the animal can quickly move away from the fearful stimulus or, if necessary, defend itself from the stimulus. In addition, the HPA response that stimulates antiproductive, antigrowth, catabolic, and immunosuppressive effects is helpful in the short-term, but if stimulated for a prolonged period or even intermittently but on a regular basis (ie, chronic intermittent stress), it results in the pathologic condition of chronic stress [17]. The immunosuppressive effects may make animals more prone to recurrent infections, and altered blood flow to various organs may make animals more susceptible to specific ailments, such as gastric ulcers [18]. Although much of the literature focuses on adrenaline, noradrenaline, and cortisol with respect to the stress response, many other neurohormones and hormones have an impact on the animal's physiologic and behavioral responses [19,20].

In short, because psychologic factors stimulate the SA system and the HPA axis, it is important to evaluate each cat not only medically in the examination room but also asking about environment, intraspecific, and interspecific interactions so as to identify potential stressors that can cause or exacerbate medical and behavioral problems.

ANXIETY AND FEAR AND HOW THEY RELATE TO SOME COMMON BEHAVIORAL PROBLEMS IN CATS

A basic understanding of the domestic cat's normal social organization can highlight the potential stressors that occur in today's typical multicat households.

Free-living domestic cats can form social groups; female kinship is suggested to be the basis of such groups [21]. The density and spatial organization of cats living in groups can vary depending on such factors as gender, reproductive status, season, and food availability. The home range of cats can vary greatly. Male cats' home range size is typically three times larger than that of females [22]. In general, however, the home range of both genders is much greater than that of most homes in which today's house cats live. Cats not belonging to the group can be the recipients of aggression from group members.

In today's households, we often have unrelated cats in small spaces with newcomers entering the space throughout the cats' life. Some cats certainly show behaviors indicative of a harmonious relationship with other cats within a house [23], whereas other cats have a difficult time adjusting to or coping with living in multicat homes.

A cat's perception of a situation influences its emotional state and, therefore, its behaviors in a situation. That cat's perception depends on a variety of factors, including but not limited to genetics, previous experience, and physiologic states (Fig. 1). Cats can have complex social relationships with other cats [23,24], but how a cat is raised in today's typical indoor environment may influence the cat's ability to cope with novel stimuli and intraspecific social relationships. Cats living outdoors in varied environments are exposed to many different stimuli, and therefore are likely to have considerably different neuropsychobiologic development compared with the typical housecat. This restricted exposure of today's typical housecat may increase their fear or anxiety about things like visitors to the home and noise fears, for example, or compromise their ability to cope in new situations [25]. Two of the more common behavioral problems related to the emotional states of fear and anxiety are intercat aggression and urine spraying [26–31].

Intercat Aggression

Fear aggression is a common form of intercat aggression. Although owners can identify overt physical fights as aggression [32], they often miss more subtle or passive forms of aggression. This is of particular concern for households in which there are no overt fights, because if a cat is distressed in an environment, it may be more likely to become inactive and inhibit many normal behaviors, including overt aggression [33]. In many cases, there may not be a clear aggressor and victim. It is not uncommon for cats to show a mixture of underlying emotions, and the main aggressor in different situations may fluctuate. Being able to identify signs of a fearful cat is crucial. Owners should be encouraged to bring in a videotape or at least point out to the clinicians pictures of what their cats look like in various situations (Figs. 2 and 3).

The specific treatment suggested depends on the specifics of each case, but categories of treatment options are as follows.

Environmental management

Environmental management varies depending on the severity of aggression and if one cat is in severe physical or emotional risk. If the risk is high, it is

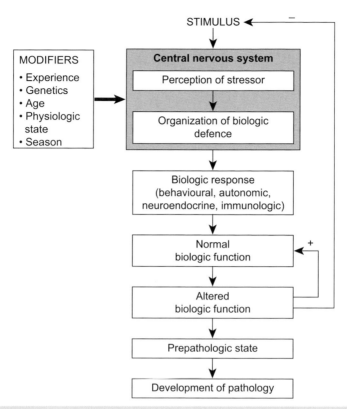

Fig. 1. Modifiers of the CNS's perception of a stressor and its organization of a biologic defense. (*Adapted from* Moberg GP. Biological response to stress: implications for animal welfare. In: Moberg GP, Mench JA, editors. The biology of animal stress. 1st edition. New York: CABI Publishing; 2000. p. 7; with permission.)

necessary to keep the cats segregated temporarily, with the exception of the times the owners are working on behavior modifications. Owners should be informed of the physical and emotional damage that could be caused by constant exposure to an aggressor without a way to alleviate that stress. Attempts at behavior modifications may be unsuccessful or at least less successful without segregation. The following suggestions are aimed at giving the cat some control over its environment. These changes may help to decrease a fear response and prevent it from turning into generalized anxiety and decrease a stress response and hopefully diminish the progression to a distress response.

- Cat shelves that accommodate one cat should be placed around the home to offer an elevated escape location for the victim or offer the aggressor a location where it is less motivated to control the other cats. By increasing vertical space in the home, the owners are effectively increasing the living space for the feline companions.

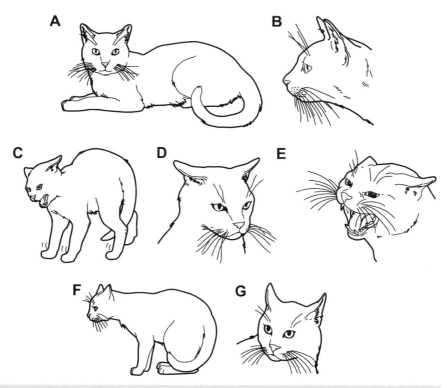

Fig. 2. (*A, B*) Alert nonthreatened cat. (*C–E*) Defensive cat. (*F, G*) Confident aggressive cat. (*Adapted from* UK Cat Behavior Working Group. An ethogram for behavioral studies of the domestic cat. UFAW Animal Welfare Research Report 8. Potters Bar (UK): Universities Federation for Animal Welfare; 1995; with permission.)

- Hide spaces, such as tunnels and cardboard boxes, around the house provide opportunities for a fearful cat to eliminate a visual source of fear or anxiety. Although we want cats to be able to hide when they are fearful, the intention is that this serves as a temporary respite. If a cat is choosing to hide most of the time, this is a red flag that the environment is not conducive to a state of good welfare and that the cat is likely experiencing generalized anxiety.
- Cat door can be installed within the home that only the victim cat has access to by wearing a magnetic collar that opens the cat door. For more open floor plans, indoor citronella invisible fencing may be an option to keep a confident aggressor out of certain rooms.
- Resource distribution: Several food and water bowl and litter box locations should be placed around the home so that the resources are dispersed. When possible, rooms with resources should have more than one entry or exit to avoid trapping a cat inside. Hiding places should also be provided in the resource room. If one cat is living in one area, that area should also have resources (litter box, food and water bowls).

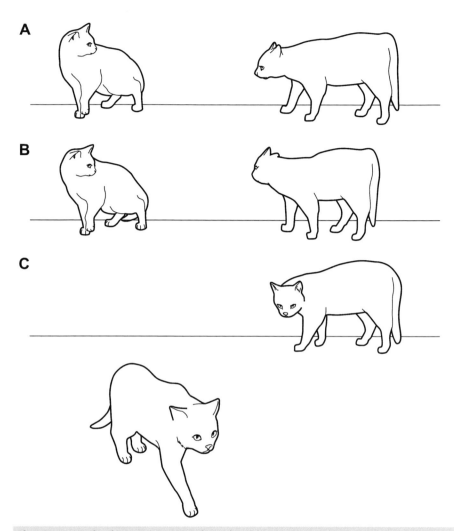

Fig. 3. (A–C) The dominant cat is on the right. The submissive cat moves slowly away and avoids eye contact. (*Adapted from* Layhausen P. Cat behavior: the predatory and social behavior of domestic and wild cats. New York: Garland STPM Press; 1979. p. 63.)

- In all cases, the aggressor should also wear an approved quick-release cat collar with a bell so that the victim is always aware of the location of the aggressor.

Environmental and cognitive enrichment
Provide the aggressor with activities that keep it mentally occupied so that it is less likely to display aggression toward the other cat(s). Some examples of various forms of enrichment to redirect the focus of the aggressor include

clicker training the aggressor, increase foraging time by teaching it how to use toys that contain their food or treats (eg, twist' n' treat; Premier Pet Products, LLC, Midlothian, Virgina), and providing cat with television by using digital versatile disks (DVDs) made specifically for cats to watch.

Behavior modification

The cornerstone of a behavioral program to help change the cats' perception of one another is a desensitization and counterconditioning (DS & CC) program. The cats are only to be exposed to one another in a minimal and controlled manner without being anxious or scared (desensitization) and to associate the other cat with positive things (counterconditioning), primarily food rewards. If this is done successfully, the cats' underlying emotional state about each other should change; therefore, the outward behavior should change as well. Owners need to be instructed to use the cat's body language (see Figs. 2 and 3) to know when to progress to the next step of the DS & CC program. Ideally, the cats would be exposed to each other in such a manner that physically safety is ensured (carriers and screen doors) and minimal aggression or anxiety is shown (ie, exposed to one another at a large distance). At this time, offering their favorite food to help them associate positive things with the presence of the other cat can be used as well. Over time, they can be brought closer together and in more realistic situations. Box 1 presents one example of a DS & CC plan. Except for the times when the owner is doing the actual behavior modifications, the cats should be kept separate from one another. Depending on the specifics of each situation, variations may need to be used on the example given. The time it takes for this to work ultimately depend on the cats involved. The author has had cases improve as quickly as a few weeks and as long as 1 year. There are some cases in which rehoming a cat or having the cats live in separate areas of the home is the only option.

Pheromones

Pheromones are naturally produced by cats and can bias behavioral and physiologic responses [34]. Feliway (Phoenix, Arizona) may be useful in cases of mild to moderate intercat aggression to help decrease anxiety. Felifriend (Chesham, England) (not yet available in the United States) may be useful when first introducing a new cat into a household but may induce a panic response when used in cases of longer term intercat aggression [35]; therefore, it is not advised as a safe form of treatment for ongoing intercat aggression at this time.

Medications

Medications commonly used for the aggressor are the tricyclic antidepressants (TCAs) and selective serotonin reuptake inhibitors (SSRIs). The reason for using the medication is to inhibit arousal levels, decrease anxious states, and improve impulse control. Once this has been done, the cat is in a state that is more conducive to behavior modifications. In the author's experience, cats seem to be more sensitive to the side effects of the TCAs as opposed to fluoxetine. Clomipramine does work on more neurotransmitters than fluoxetine [36]

Box 1: Example of a desensitization and counterconditioning plan for intercat aggression within a home

Stage 1 concept

Desensitize and then countercondition the cats to each other's scent.

> Stage 1 implementation: Take a washcloth/unscented tissue and rub it on the cheeks of the victim cat and let the aggressor smell it. Watch for bodily reaction, such as hissing, spitting, tail swishing, fluffing, and ears back. Do this at least twice day until the reaction decreases; at that time, pair the smelling of the cloth with feeding of the cat's favorite food.
>
> Stage 1 implementation: Rotate the cats' litter boxes without completely cleaning them.

Stage 2 concept

Once the cat has been desensitized and counterconditioned to the scent of the other cat, start DS & CC to the sight of the other cat.

> Stage 2 implementation: Put each cat into a large carrier and place them at a large enough distance away from each other so there are minimal if any signs of aggression. Feed each cat its favorite food at this time. Once the cats are done eating, put cats back into their respective areas of the home. These sessions should be short and positive. If no aggression is shown, continue for several days and then start moving the carriers closer to one another in small increments (eg, 6 inches). Repeat exercises until the cats can be relatively close without showing signs of fear and aggression and are willing to eat or play with a toy (whatever reward works for the cat).

Stage 3 concept

Once the cats are desensitized and counterconditioned to the sight of one another, we need to start getting them used to a more natural setting slowly.

> Stage 3 implementation: You can let the victim out of the carrier and walk around, because the aggressor is still in the carrier and continue to pair this with rewarding the aggressor.
>
> Stage 3 implementation: You can use a screen door inside the house to keep cats separate but allow them to see each other walk, approach, and sniff, for example, and pair with rewards.
>
> Stage 3 implementation: You may need to use a harness on the aggressor when first allowing that cat out of the carrier and pair bringing cats to gether with rewards.
>
> Stage 3 implementation: You can keep a door in your home slightly ajar so that the cats cannot become aggressive but can touch paws if they so choose.

Stage 4 concept

If no aggression is shown with allowing them more freedom during the aforementioned controlled short exercises, the cats can be brought together for short supervised sessions in the home setting as long as other modalities (environmental and medications) have been implemented as mentioned in the article.

and can decrease arousal levels pretty dramatically; in certain cases of intercat aggression, this may prove useful. To avoid oversedation, it is advised that the dose be started out at the lowest suggested dose and titrated up as needed every 3 to 6 weeks. If impulse control is more of the concern, fluoxetine would be useful in that it blocks reuptake of serotonin, as does clomipramine, but does not have the high side effect profile of clomipramine. One should consider medicating the victim as well if the victim is experiencing considerable anxiety. Anxiety can be expressed with overt behaviors like continual hiding; hypervigilance; becoming withdrawn; and changes in appetite, sleep patterns, and sociability. Caution should be used in using benzodiazepines because these may disinhibit aggression but may be appropriate for victims whose behaviors are hiding and running without any aggression. Buspirone is another option for victims that do not respond with aggression; however, this medication may boost the confidence of the victim, who may then react with aggression. All medications used for intercat aggression or anxiety are off-label. Medications are typically used in cats that are showing affective aggression, which is the focus of this article, but it is important to note that for cats appearing to be aggressing in a normal sociobiologic way (calm confident body postures and territorial in nature), medication may be helpful, but it is important to realize that the cat may be acting in a very "normal" manner that is simply not acceptable to the owner. In these cases, owners need to be made aware of this and prepared for a guarded prognosis, and they must consider the ethics and welfare of medicating this cat and allowing the other cats to be continually victimized in the home. In cases of territorial aggression, it may be more humane for all involved to rehome the territorial cat to a single-cat household or to have the owners permanently segregate the cats within their home.

Urine Spraying

Urine spraying is a normal behavior in male and female cats. Although the ethologic basis for spraying is not well known, several reasons why our domestic cats may spray have been postulated [37–40], in which fear, anxiety, stress, and distress may be included.

Urine marks are usually found on vertical surfaces, and the location of the marks within the home can provide information about the cause of marking (Box 2). Treatment should focus on the suspected underlying cause of spraying. For cases revolving around fear and anxiety, the following treatment options are recommended.

Treatment

Every effort should be made to identify triggers so that a DS & CC plans can be implemented. Cats should be provided with environmental options as mentioned previously to provide them some control over their environment so that they can choose to remove themselves from the source of fear. Pheromone therapy (Feliway) can be used to reduce the incidence of spraying; however, if the spraying is a direct result of overt intercat aggression within the home, the pheromone therapy may not be as effective. [41–44]. Frank and colleagues [41]

Box 2: Indoor marking patterns

- Initial locations around cat flap, external doors, and windows: external threat
- Initial locations are entry points to internal rooms, on landings, and in corridors: internal conflict within a home
- Spread of marking sights into the home from around the cat flap: potential intruder cat
- Random locations throughout the home: emotional disturbance within the household
- Initial deposits on new items in the household, shoes, or shopping bags: insecurity and reaction to potential threat

From Bowen B, Heath S. Behavior problems in the small animal. Philadelphia: Elsevier; 2005; with permission.

found that in homes in which the spraying occurred with overt intercat aggression, the Feliway was not as efficacious. This is not too surprising, given that pheromones are a form of chemical communication to help signal the animal that there is no need to be anxious or stressed; however, if the victim cat is being visually threatened by another cat in the house, it is unlikely that a subtle chemical cue would override such a strong visual cue. Another strategy is to try and encourage the cat to mark the area by using its cheek glands as opposed to urine. Owners can do this by placing cat combs (Mr Spats Cat-A-Comb) around the house in areas where their cats are likely to mark. Adding more scratching posts may also encourage a cat to mark with its claws if it is a cat that currently uses scratching posts. One study found that by adding more litter boxes, increasing litter box cleanliness, and cleaning urine marks with an enzymatic cleaner, the incidence of spraying was reduced [45]. In areas frequently marked, a litter box can be placed vertically to minimize damage to the house and make cleaning up easier. Resources, such as food and water, should be spread out so that the cats do not need to congregate in close proximity. If the stimulus causing the cat to spray is outside, clients can use privacy paper to cover the windows and, if possible, attempt to get the outdoor cat to stay away. Privacy paper allows for the visual acuity to be decreased but permits sunlight into the home.

Psychoactive medication may be needed to help relieve anxiety, especially in cases in which there are no clearly identifiable triggers or when owners are unable to make behavior and or environmental modifications. For clients demanding fast results, a benzodiazepine can be used in conjunction with a TCA or SSRI. After a few weeks, if the spraying has decreased, the benzodiazepine can be tapered off. Drug dosages used in spraying are presented in Table 1. A recent study on clomipramine's efficacy for spraying found that without any changes in the environment or any behavior modifications, clomipramine alone (0.54 mg/kg administered orally once daily) reduced the

Table 1
Drug therapy for urine marking in cats

Drug	Dosage	Comments
Clomipramine	0.3–0.5 mg/kg q 24 h (2.5–5 mg per cat q 24 h)	Mild anticholinergic; 80% or more of cats improved; no placebo trial; greater than 50% recurrence when drug withdrawn
Amitriptyline	0.5–1 mg/kg q 24 h (approximately 2.5–5 mg per cat q 24 h)	Anticholinergic; highly bitter; no published trials
Fluoxetine	0.5–1 mg/kg q 24 h (2.5–5 mg per cat q 24 h)	Significant improvement over placebo in small trial
Paroxetine	0.5–1 mg/kg q 24 h (2.5–5 mg per cat q 24 h)	Mild anticholinergic effects
Buspirone	2.5–7.5 mg per cat q 12 h	Expensive; minimal side effects; twice daily dosing; 55% improved, 50% recurrence on withdrawal
Diazepam	1–2.5 mg per cat q 24 or 12 h	Potential for hepatotoxicity; up to 75% improvement; up to 90% recurrence on withdrawal; may cause ataxia, sedation, appetite increase
Oxazepam	0.2–1 mg/kg per cat q 24 or 12 h	No clinical trials; may be less potential for hepatotoxicity than diazepam
Selegiline	0.5–1 mg/kg per cat q 24 h	May be useful in cognitive dysfunction or for more generalized emotional disorders
Megestrol acetate	5 mg per cat q 24 h for 2 wk, then wean slowly to lowest effective maintenance dose	Poor efficacy (50% neutered males, 10% spayed females); potential for numerous side effects
Medroxyprogesterone	5–20 mg/kg subcutaneous q 4 or more mo	May be less effective than megestrol; injectable formulation; potential for numerous side effects

Abbreviation: q, every.

From Landsberg G, Hunthausen W, Ackerman L. Handbook of behavior problems of the dog and cat. Philadelphia: Elsevier; 2003. p. 375; with permission.

incidence of spraying by approximately 75% in 20 of 25 cats within 4 weeks [46]. Another study compared the efficacy of fluoxetine and clomipramine and found that both medications were equivalent in treating spraying behavior in cats. Treatment longer than 8 weeks revealed a higher rate of a reduced incidence of spraying, and although the spraying was likely to return if the medication was abruptly discontinued, reinstatement of the original medication was just as efficacious in reducing the spraying as it was the first time [47]. While waiting for the TCA or SSRI to take effect, clients can try using piddle pants if the cat tolerates wearing them, or they may be useful in cases in which medication is not an option. Punishment, verbal or physical, is never appropriate and can make the problem worse. Enzymatic cleaners are recommended to clean up soiled areas, and the owners should be encouraged to try various brands.

When drugs are used as part of a treatment program for behavior problems, the author suggests that practitioners read the article and any listed references in the article by Seibert and Landsberg elsewhere in this issue. For those drugs that are not licensed for veterinary use, doses, indications, side effects, and contraindications may not be adequately studied. Practitioners should be familiar with the published literature and dispense these medications with informed consent.

SUMMARY

Emotions can no longer be dismissed as irrelevant or inconsequential in animals. Emotions play a significant role in how animals behave and in stimulating the stress response. Treatment plans should focus on how to reduce the emotional states of anxiety and fear. By doing this, we, as veterinarians, are improving the state of welfare for these animals and safeguarding not only their mental well-being but their physical well-being.

References

[1] McMillan FD. Stress, distress, and emotion: distinctions and implications for mental well-being. In: McMillan FD, editor. Mental health and well-being in animals. Iowa (IA): Blackwell; 2005. p. 93–125.
[2] Buffington CA, Westropp JL, Chew DJ, et al. Clinical evaluation of multimodal environmental modification (MEMO) in the management of cats with idiopathic cystitis. J Feline Med Surg 2006;8:261–8.
[3] Forrester SD, Roudebush P. Evidence based management of feline lower urinary tract disease. Vet Clin North Am Small Anim Pract 2007;37(3):533–58.
[4] Cameron ME, Casey RA, Bradshaw JWS, et al. A study of environmental and behavioral factors that may be associated with feline idiopathic cystitis. J Small Anim Pract 2004;45:144–7.
[5] Moberg GP. Biological response to stress: implications for animal welfare. In: Moberg GP, Mench JA, editors. The biology of animal stress. 1st edition. New York: CABI Publishing; 2000. p. 1–21.
[6] Casey R. Fear and stress. In: Horwitz D, Mills D, Heath S, editors. BSAVA manual of canine and feline behavioural medicine. 1st edition. Gloucester (UK): BSAVA; 2002. p. 144–53.
[7] Öhman A. In: Lewis M, Haviand-Jones J, editors. Handbook of emotions. 2nd edition. New York: The Guilford Press; 2000. p. 573–93.

[8] Kitchen H, Arosnon AL, Bittel JL, et al. Panel report on the colloquium on recognition and alleviation of animal pain and distress. J Am Vet Med Assoc 1987;191:1186–91.

[9] Singer J. Sympathetic activation, drugs, and fear. J Comp Physiol Psychol 1963;56:612–5.

[10] Haroutunian V, Riccio DC. Effect of arousal conditions during restraint treatment upon learned fear in young rats. Dev Psychobiol 1977;10:25–32.

[11] Bear MF, Connors BW, Paradiso MA. Mental illness. In: Katz S, editor. Neuroscience exploring the brain. Maryland (MD): Lippincott Williams & Wilkins; 2001. p. 675–701.

[12] Clark JD, Rager DR, Calpin JP. Animal well-being. II. Stress and distress. Lab Anim Sci 2005;47:571–9.

[13] Mason JW. Emotion as reflected in patterns of endocrine integration. In: Levi L, editor. Emotions: their parameters and measurement. New York: Raven Press; 2007. p.143–81.

[14] Mason JW, Maher JT, Hartley LH, et al. Selectivity of corticosteroid and catecholamine responses to various natural stimuli. In: Serban G, editor. Psychopathology of human adaption. New York: Plenum Press; 1976. p. 147–71.

[15] Moberg GP. Problems defining stress and distress in animals. J Am Vet Med Assoc 1987;191:1207–11.

[16] Le Moal M, Simon H. Mesocorticolimbic dopaminergic network: functional and regulatory roles. Physiol Rev 1991;71:155–234.

[17] Ladewig J. Chronic intermittent stress: a model for the study of long-term stressors. In: Moberg GP, Mench JA, editors. The biology of animal stress. 1st edition. New York: CABI Publishing; 2000. p. 159–69.

[18] Sapolsky RM. Ulcers, the runs, and hot fudge sundays. In: Why zebras don't get ulcers. 4th edition. New York: Henry Holt & Co; 2004. p. 71–91.

[19] Sapolsky RM. Glands, gooseflesh, and hormones. In: Why zebras don't get ulcers. 4th edition. New York: Henry Holt & Co; 2004. p. 19–36.

[20] Matteri RL, Carroll JA, Dyer CJ. Neuroendocrine responses to stress. In: Moberg GP, Mench JA, editors. The biology of animal stress. 1st edition. New York: CABI Publishing; 2000. p. 43–76.

[21] MacDonald DW. The social behavior of a group of semi-independent farm cats, felis catus: a progress report. Carnivore Genetic Newsletter 1978;3:256–68.

[22] Libers O, Sandell M, Pontier D, et al. Density, spatial organization, and reproductive tactics in the domestic cat and other felids. In: Turner DC, Bateson P, editors. The domestic cat. 2nd edition. Cambridge (UK): Cambridge University Press; 2000. p. 120–47.

[23] Curtis TM, Knowles RJ, Crowell-Davis SL. Influence of familiarity and relatedness on proximity and allogrooming in domestic cats (felis catus). Am J Vet Res 2003;64(9):1151–4.

[24] Macdonald DW, Yamaguchi N, Kerby G. Group-living in the domestic cat: its sociobiology and epidemiology. In: Turner DC, Bateson P, editors. The domestic cat: the biology of its behavior. 2nd edition. Cambridge (UK): Cambridge University Press; 2000. p. 96–118.

[25] Mason WA. Early developmental influences of experience on behaviour, temperament and stress. In: Moberg GP, Mench JA, editors. The biology of animal stress. 1st edition. New York: CABI Publishing; 2000. p. 269–90.

[26] Beaver BV. Housesoiling by cats: a retrospective study of 120 cases. J Am Vet Med Assoc 1989;25:631–7.

[27] Borchelt PL, Voith VL. Elimination behavior problems in cats. Compendium on Continuing Education for the Practicing Veterinarian 1986;8:197–207.

[28] Olm DD, Houpt KA. Feline house-soiling problems. Appl Anim Behav Sci 1988;20:335–45.

[29] Borchelt PL, Voith VL. Aggressive behavior in cats. In: Voith VL, Borchelt PL, editors. Readings in companion animal behavior. Trenton (NJ): Veterinary Learning Systems; 1996. p. 208–16.

[30] Heidenberger E. Housing conditions and behavioural problems of indoor cats as assessed by their owners. Appl Anim Behav Sci 1997;52:345–64.

[31] Houpt KA. Aggression and social structure. In: Domestic animal behavior for veterinarians and animal scientists. 3rd edition. Iowa (IA): Iowa State Univ Press; 1998. p. 33–81.

[32] Levine E, Perry P, Scarlett J, et al. Intercat aggression in households following the introduction of a new cat. Appl Anim Behav Sci 2004;90:325–36.

[33] Rochlitz I. Feline welfare issues. In: Turner DC, Bateson P, editors. The domestic cat: the biology of its behavior. 2nd edition. Cambridge (UK): Cambridge University Press; 2000. p. 208–26.

[34] Kelliher KR. The combined role of the main olfactory and vomeronasal systems in social communication in mammals. Horm Behav 2007;52:561–70.

[35] Heath S. Feline aggression. In: Horwitz D, Mills D, Heath S, editors. BSAVA manual of canine and feline behavioural medicine. 1st edition. Gloucester (UK): BSAVA; 2002. p. 216–28.

[36] Stahl SM. Classical antidepressants, serotonin selective reuptake inhibitors, and noradrenergic reuptake inhibitors. In: Essential psychopharmacology. 2nd edition. Cambridge (UK): Cambridge University Press; 2000. p. 199–243.

[37] Simpson BS. Feline house-soiling. Part II: urine and fecal marking. Compendium on Continuing Education for the Practicing Veterinarian 1998;20:331–9.

[38] Dehasse J. Feline urine spraying. Appl Anim Behav Sci 1997;52:365–71.

[39] Borchelt PL. Cat elimination problems. Vet Clin North Am Small Anim Pract 1991;2(2): 254–65.

[40] Natoli E, De Vito E. Agonistic behavior, dominance rank and copulatory success in large multi-male feral cat, felis catus, colony in central Rome. Anim Behav 1991;42:227–41.

[41] Frank DF, Erb HN, Houpt KA. Urine spraying in cats: presence of concurrent disease and effects of a pheromone treatment. Appl Anim Behav Sci 1999;61:263–72.

[42] Mills DS, Mills CB. Evaluation of a novel method for delivering a synthetic analogue of feline facial pheromone to control urine spraying by cats. Vet Rec 2001;149:197–9.

[43] Mills DS, White JC. Long-term follow up of the effect of a pheromone therapy on feline spraying behavior. Vet Rec 2000;147:746–7.

[44] Hunthausen W. Evaluating a feline facial pheromone analogue to control urine spraying. Vet Med 2000 Feb;151–5.

[45] Pryor PA, Hart BL, Bain MJ, et al. Causes of urine marking in cats and the effects of environmental management on the frequency of marking. J Am Vet Med Assoc 2001;219: 1709–13.

[46] Landsberg GM, Wilson AL. Effect of clomipramine in cats presented for urine marking. J Am Anim Hosp Assoc 2005;41:3–11.

[47] Hart BL, Cliff KD, Tynes VV, et al. Control of urine marking by use of long term treatment with fluoxetine or clomipramine in cats. J Am Vet Med Assoc 2005;226(3):378–82.

Vet Clin Small Anim 38 (2008) 1081–1106

VETERINARY CLINICS
SMALL ANIMAL PRACTICE

Canine Anxieties and Phobias: An Update on Separation Anxiety and Noise Aversions

Barbara L. Sherman, PhD, DVM[a],*,
Daniel S. Mills, BVSc, PhD, CBiol, MIBiol, CCAB, MRCVS[b]

[a]Department of Clinical Sciences, North Carolina State University College of Veterinary Medicine, 4700 Hillsborough Street, Raleigh, NC 27606–1499, USA
[b]Department of Biological Sciences, University of Lincoln, Riseholme Park, Lincoln, LN2 2LG, UK

F or many dogs, the world is a fearful place, particularly when left alone or when subjected to disturbing sounds. On a daily basis, many dogs that live as companions to people experience anxiety states so severe that they crush door knobs with their teeth or catapult themselves through plate-glass windows in an apparent attempt to reunite with their owners. These dogs are experiencing separation anxiety. Other companion dogs pant, pace, and tremble when subjected to anxiety-producing sounds, such as thunderstorms. These dogs are experiencing noise aversions. The intensity of these responses is in marked contrast to the nonproblematic behavior of many of these dogs, described as "stable in temperament" [1]. This apparent contradiction can puzzle and frustrate owners and veterinarians alike as they struggle to manage such cases. Separation anxiety and noise aversions affect the welfare of the affected dog and the stability of the human-animal bond. Even the most dedicated owner is taxed by observing the dog's distress and experiencing the financial and emotion cost of destructiveness, house soiling, or other secondary problem behaviors. This article focuses on two common problems relating to fearful states of dogs: separation anxiety and noise aversions.

There is overlap between the definition and common use of the terms *anxiety*, *fear*, and *phobia*, although the underlying neural and emotional systems may be different. Anxiety is a reaction to a prospective or imagined danger or uncertainty. Anxiety includes physiologic signs (eg, increased respiratory and heart rates, vasomotor changes, trembling or paralysis, increased salivation or sweating, gastrointestinal disturbances) and behavioral signs. The behavioral signs may include changes in activity (eg, immobility, pacing, circling, restlessness);

*Corresponding author. Department of Clinical Sciences, North Carolina State University College of Veterinary Medicine, 4700 Hillsborough Street, Raleigh, NC 27606–1499. *E-mail address*: barbara_sherman@ncsu.edu (B.L. Sherman).

0195-5616/08/$ – see front matter
doi:10.1016/j.cvsm.2008.04.012

changes in nearest neighbor distances (eg, remaining close to a person or conspecific); or changes in appetite, including anorexia.

Fear is an emotion of alarm and agitation caused by a present or threatened danger. Among animals, fear is manifest by physiologic responses, such as tachycardia, hypersalivation, or elimination, in addition to behavioral responses associated with escape, avoidance, or defensiveness. Fear responses occur in response to the presence or proximity of an object, individual, or social situation.

A phobia is a marked, persistent, and excessive fear of clearly discernible circumscribed objects or situations. Exposure to a phobic stimulus almost invariably provokes an immediate behavioral response with concomitant physiological signs of autonomic arousal. The response may take the form of a situationally bound or situationally predisposed "panic attack." Phobias often lead to avoidance behavior.

In clinical practice, these semantic distinctions and their underlying neural and emotional correlates are ambiguous. It has become conventional to refer to all manifestations of separation distress or frustration as "separation anxiety," although some dogs may be minimally anxious and others experience what is likened to a panic attack. Similarly, certain sounds may elicit responses consistent with anxious or phobic responses. Herein, the term *noise aversion* is used to refer to all anxious, fearful, and phobic responses to sounds.

SEPARATION ANXIETY

Canine separation anxiety is a behavioral disorder of dogs when left alone or separated from a significant person or persons. The term *separation distress* may best describe the phenomenon, which incorporates signs consistent with anxiety, fear, and phobic behavior. Separation anxiety is manifest by several behavioral signs, including destructiveness, rearrangement of household objects, hypersalivation, inappropriate urination and defecation (in a dog otherwise well house trained), distress vocalization, restlessness, and other signs [2–5].

Separation anxiety is common. Several telephone marketing surveys of pet owners in the United States reveal that signs of separation anxiety occur in approximately 14% (Allpoints Research, Winston-Salem, North Carolina, 1997) and 17% (Lilly Market Research, Greenfield, Indiana, 2006) of owned dogs that receive veterinary care. In the United Kingdom, at least 20% of dogs are believed to have separation anxiety [6], although up to 50% of dogs in the population may display clinical signs at some time [7]. Separation anxiety cases make up 20% to 40% of the caseloads of behavior specialty practices [8–10].

Separation anxiety has an erosive effect on the human-animal bond. The disorder often appears in dogs that have high emotional value to their owners. In fact, clients often report that their dogs are "perfect 95% of the time," emphasizing the positive qualities of the relationship with their pet and allocating a relatively small percent of time to the behavior problem. When the problem results in hundreds or thousands of dollars of damage to the home or is a focus of marital disharmony in a family, however, the remaining 5% is magnified. People, in addition to dogs, experience distress and frustration, especially when destruction is prominent [11] or the offending dog is resistant to treatment. The owner's conflict over his or her attachment to the dog, on the one hand, and the emotional and monetary cost of the disorder, on the other hand, may irreparably erode the human-animal bond and result in rehoming, relinquishment to an animal shelter [12–15], or even euthanasia of the offending dog [17]. The paradox between the attachment of the owner to the dog and the breaking of the human-animal bond is a common theme in the evaluation of cases of separation anxiety [18].

ETIOLOGIC FACTORS

There are several factors reported to be associated with canine separation anxiety. These include a history of long periods of being left alone, long periods with the owner without being left alone, periods of kennel housing [8], shelter housing [3,8,19], family move to new house or apartment [10,20], urban housing [10], and loss of a family pet [10]. In one study, dogs from a home with a single adult owner were approximately 2.5 times more likely to exhibit signs of separation distress as dogs from a home with multiple owners [21]. In another study, households comprised of couples with children were overrepresented [21]. Singleton owners may report that they often stay home after work and eschew social engagements to avoid leaving their dogs alone for additional periods (Barbara L. Sherman, personal observations, 2006–2008). Clients may report to the clinician feelings of guilt for working and leaving dogs alone for long periods and may compensate with excessive attention during time together.

Separation anxiety may be a disorder of our times and our lifestyles: single-individual households [20], long owner work days [10], restricted interdog social opportunities, and limited exercise may predispose animals to separation distress. Because it may not be possible to correct underlying environmental factors, treatment of the dog becomes imperative, simultaneously to improve its welfare and to salvage the human-animal bond. As our lives become more solitary and compartmentalized, the role of dogs as social companions may become increasingly important [18].

Numerous factors may underly the expression of separation anxiety; a recent multifactorial explanation for separation anxiety has been proposed [22]. One causal factor may be heritable, because some experienced owners of purebred dogs with separation anxiety anecdotally report that, contrary to unaffected puppies, the affected puppy "never 'got over' usual weaning distress" (BL Sherman, personal observation, 1996–2007). Many dogs that exhibit separation anxiety have been adopted from an animal shelter or through rescue routes, and their early history is unknown. It is possible that these dogs never recovered from weaning distress or that they were the offspring of dogs that themselves exhibited separation distress. Alternately, it is possible that the early experiences of these dogs predisposed them to the behavioral disorder.

SHERMAN & MILLS

Inadequate socialization, juvenile illness, or an anxious or ambivalent dam may be at-risk factors for behavior problems, including separation distress [19]. Excessive human social interactions after adoption and subsequent withdrawal of social interaction when left alone may sensitize dogs to departures [3,7]. It is also possible that dogs with separation anxiety may "revolve" through animal shelters, repeatedly adopted and relinquished.

The attachment of the owner to the dog and dog to the owner, in excess termed *hyperattachment*, is widely debated in the literature on separation anxiety [22]. Clinically, dogs that follow their owners when home and seek constant physical contact are commonly presented with a diagnosis of separation anxiety. Not all cases present such signs of hyperattachment, however, and it is not a necessary criterion for an operational diagnosis of separation anxiety. Explanations for hyperattachment are disparate, such as the result of retention of neotenic characteristics secondary to domestication [19] or a response shaped by the owner's behavior, reinforcing attention-seeking, physical contact, and following behaviors [22].

The heterogeneity of cases presented for separation distress has stimulated investigation into other causal factors. In the 1990s, based on the observation that many dogs with separation distress retained juvenile behavioral characteristics, it was theorized that separation anxiety resulted from behavioral neoteny, the retention of juvenile characteristics, including attachment [23]. An explanation was needed for dogs that demonstrated signs of separation anxiety but did not exhibit hyperattachment, however.

A refined model was proposed by Appleby and Pluijmakers [22] that describes three types of separation distress, designated class A, B, and C. Case evaluation and statistical analysis have supported this schema.

Dogs assigned to class A exhibit primary hyperattachment to the owner. During development, these dogs retain puppy-like behavior patterns, including oral exploration. They form rapid, strong, and excessive attachment to a specific person, generally the owner, and exhibit characteristic responses to the departure of this person. When the owner picks up his or her keys or puts on a coat in preparation for departure, class A dogs become increasingly anxious. When left alone, such dogs may attempt reunion by digging or chewing doors and howl or otherwise vocalize using long-range communication signals apparently to recruit the owner. When the owner returns home, the dog shows intense and protracted greeting.

Dogs assigned to class B exhibit secondary hyperattachment. They appear normal as puppies. Their emotional attachment to a particular individual, another animal, or even an inanimate object develops later in life than the dogs in class A. This may coincide with a change in circumstances, such as a move to a new house or increased time spent with the owner when he or she is at home ill. In the absence of the owner, these dogs may orient toward objects associated with the owner's scent, such as the television remote control. These dogs have the potential to substitute one individual for another and may be comforted by familiar objects or locations.

Dogs assigned to class C develop separation distress at any age in response to a fearful or unpleasant event or events, such as a thunderstorm, which occur when the owner is absent, resulting in a conditioned fear of isolation. The owner may be unaware of this learned association, particularly based on retrospective recall. In general, these dogs are generally well adapted and show few signs of hyperattachment, except when exposed to the fearful stimulus in the presence of the owner. For example, if the fearful stimulus is a thunderstorm, the dog may show some anxiety in response to thunderstorms even with the owner present, or the owner may be able to calm the animal completely. The associated separation-related signs may be sporadic and may be related more to panic than to an attempt to reunite with the owner. The dog may seek a safe place by digging or may "disarrange" furnishings or damage immoveable objects.

In one study that compared 200 dogs with separation anxiety with 200 control dogs, there was no association between spoiling activities (feeding the dog from the table or allowing the dog on the owner's bed) and separation anxiety [20,24]. Other studies have suggested a decreased incidence of behavior problems, including separation anxiety, in dogs that have had obedience training [25,26].

Separation anxiety has an environmental component, possibly based on familiarity. In one study, adult dogs under conditions of social isolation produced distress barking only in a familiar environment. When isolated in an unfamiliar environment, distress vocalizations were inhibited [27]. This may explain why some dogs with separation distress can be left alone in a car without vocalizing [8].

In other cases, dogs not trained to crate confinement tolerate being left alone loose in the house but display separation distress when restricted to a crate [28]. In fact, many dogs confined to a crate to prevent destruction of the house and exhibiting bar biting and hypersalivation in the crate, continue to improve when successfully treated even when left out of the crate. For these dogs, a treatment goal is to manage them successfully so that crate confinement is not necessary. In one study, 12% of 242 dogs with separation anxiety were confined to a crate during the absence of the owner [5].

SIGNALMENT

In some studies of separation anxiety, there is a gender bias toward male dogs [8,10,17,20,29]. In other studies, both genders are approximately equally represented [5,30,31]. Some of the latter studies were large clinical trials [5,30], which excluded from participation dogs that exhibited human-directed aggression. Thus, dogs with separation anxiety that were aggressive toward owners in an apparent attempt to prevent their imminent departure may have been excluded from the study population. Because owner-directed aggression is more common in male dogs, more male dogs may have been excluded than female dogs from the study population, resulting in a gender ratio biased toward parity.

No specific breed category seems to be overrepresented consistently with regard to separation anxiety, except mixed-breed dogs. The relative percentages of purebred dogs versus mixed-breed dogs diagnosed with the disorder range from study to study. When compared with representation in the general population in one study, no bias was observed [7]. Purebred dogs comprise 48% [17] to 67% [8] of the study populations. Mixed-breed dogs make up the remainder, ranging from 33% [8] to 52% [17]. The representation of mixed-breed dogs is not independent of source, because in many studies, dogs obtained from shelters or rescue are overrepresented and mixed-breed dogs are overrepresented in shelter populations. Purebred dogs tend to be obtained from breeders. In one study, 26% of dogs presented to a university teaching hospital for separation anxiety were adopted from animal shelters versus 8% of dogs presented to the same hospital for medical or surgical reasons [8].

Age of first manifestation of clinical signs of the affected animal shows a wide range. Because all puppies experience some separation distress during the weaning period [22] and juveniles exhibit destructive play behavior [11] in addition to inadequate housetraining, a diagnosis of separation anxiety is generally not definitively made until the age of 6 months. In some cases, however, purebred dogs presented for persistent separation anxiety have failed to recover from normal separation distress at weaning, suggesting to experienced dog owners a heritable component to separation anxiety in these individuals. Such historical information is often unknown in dogs obtained after puppyhood.

DIAGNOSIS

A diagnosis of separation anxiety can be made on the basis of a thorough behavioral history and medical evaluation [9,22] to rule out medical differential diagnoses and behavioral differential diagnoses (Table 1). Medical evaluations are especially important in cases of elimination in an otherwise housetrained dog and in geriatric patients. The behavioral history is imperative to confirm the diagnosis of separation anxiety and to rule out other behavioral differential diagnoses (see Table 1).

The behavioral diagnosis of separation anxiety should be considered if there are signs only when the owner is gone. These may include destruction at doors of egress, apparently random destruction in the home, or other destruction when the owner is gone [11]. The most obvious clinical determinants of separation anxiety are findings by the owner on return that include destruction (general or restricted to doors or windows), disarrangement of objects in the household, inappropriate urination or defecation in an otherwise well–housetrained dog, excessive salivation, or distress vocalization that can be heard by listening outside after stealthy return or by neighbors. In a recent study of 242 dogs whose diagnosis was confirmed by a board-certified veterinary behaviorist, 80.2% displayed destructiveness or rearrangement, 35.1% displayed inappropriate urination, 27.6% displayed inappropriate defecation, and 33.4% exhibited hypersalivation [5]. It should be emphasized that for a simple

Table 1
Medical and behavioral differential diagnoses for signs consistent with separation anxiety

Sign in absence of significant person	Medical differentials for clinical signs	Behavioral differentials for clinical signs
Destruction or rearranging	Hepatic encephalopathy	Playful behavior Puppy chewing Thunderstorm or noise phobia Territorial aggression Overactivity (inadequate exercise, exploration, arousal) Cognitive dysfunction
Inappropriate urination	Cystitis, other disorders of the lower urinary tract	Inadequate housetraining
	Diabetes; endocrine or neoplastic disorders that increase urine volume	Inadequate opportunity (inadequate urinary bladder capacity, excessive departure time, inadequate availability of suitable elimination sites)
	Seizures	Submissive/greeting/excitement Urine marking Fear-induced (noise, other) Cognitive dysfunction
Inappropriate defecation	Gastrointestinal disease (colitis, parasites)	Inadequate housetraining
	Dietary (high-bulk diet, dietary sensitivity, or allergies)	Inadequate opportunity (excessive departure time of owner, inadequate availability of suitable elimination sites
	Seizures	Cognitive dysfunction
Hypersalivation	Toxin exposure	
Excessive distress vocalization	Hepatic encephalopathy	Territorial behavior or aggression to outside stimuli Social communication (inside or outside stimuli) Play Thunderstorm or noise phobia Reaction to arousing stimuli
Self-trauma	Hepatic encephalopathy Acral lick dermatitis Allergic dermatitis Neuritis Other dermatologic disorder Parasites	Canine compulsive disorder Play

Data from Refs. [3,8,9,11,23].

diagnosis of separation anxiety, these behaviors should not occur at times when the owner is at home.

Detection of other common signs of separation anxiety, such as restlessness, pacing, circling, or panting, may require videotaping capture in the owner's absence [32]. An audio recorder may be used to document vocalizations and a cardiac monitor attached to the dog may be used to record cardiac responses.

Social conditions should be considered. Dogs with hyperattachment may exhibit separation anxiety when the owner or specific attachment figure is absent and show little comfort by the presence of other individuals. In the absence of the owner, other dogs may accept familiar individuals as acceptable substitutes and express distress only when left alone.

Behavioral signs when the owner is home may encompass hyperattachment, including attention seeking, physical contact, following, and distress on exclusion from visual contact with the owner. When preparing to depart, the dog may display signs consistent with anxiety, such as panting or pacing, or mimic a state of catatonia, seeking a site of refuge and not moving. The dog's appetite during this period and when the owner is gone may be diminished or absent. As the owner departs, some dogs exhibit aggression, often directed at the feet or hands, in an apparent attempt to prevent egress. These dogs may represent a special subset of separation distress [22]. It should be noted that aggression toward people was an exclusion criterion from several large studies of pharmacologic agents approved for the treatment of separation anxiety. On the owner's return home, the affected dog may exhibit excessive duration and intensity of greeting that persists beyond reasonable expectation.

TREATMENT

Separation anxiety should be treated immediately. Households with dogs experiencing this disorder are in distress because of the emotional hardship of watching a dog suffer daily and the financial cost of destructiveness and house soiling. Because one family member may advocate for the dog, whereas another may advocate for the household budget, the condition can lead to rancor within the household and eviction of the dog.

Treatment consists of owner education, environmental management, behavior modification techniques, and administration of therapeutic agents (behavioral drugs and pheromones). Owner education is extremely important. Often, owners attribute the dog's misbehavior to spite, do not understand canine social communication, and do not understand behavior modification techniques [4]. The purpose of environmental management is to reduce manifestation of signs and reduce strain in the household to permit time for behavior modification and pharmacotherapy to become effective.

Treatment success may depend on the presenting signs and the interactions with the owner. It is useful to customize treatment based on the subtype of separation anxiety displayed by each affected animal [22]. Improved treatment success may be obtained by specifically diagnosing the subtype of separation anxiety and targeting treatment to that subtype [22]. For those dogs in class

A, hyperattached, treatment is directed toward reducing dependence on the owner or the individual to whom the dog is hyperattached and also treating the secondary problems. Those dogs in class B do not display hyperattachment. The primary aim of treatment in class B cases should be to focus on restoring comfort stimuli and things that actually help the animal to relax; as substitutes are found, the animal becomes better able to cope with being left alone. Examples of inanimate objects that dogs may become attached to might be something like an indoor kennel or crate or a blanket associated with the owner's scent. For those dogs in class C, behavior treatment needs to focus on helping the animal to cope with its underlying fear rather than the attachment to the owner [22].

Environmental Management

If at all possible, in the initial stages of treatment, the dog's exposure to the situation that provokes anxiety should be minimized or eliminated. For example, rather than being left alone at home, the dog can be dropped off for day boarding while the owner is gone. This prevents recurrences of extreme anxiety that perpetuate conditioned responses. It also immediately reduces manifestation of clinical signs that upset the household. When left alone at home, to avoid destructiveness in the house, a safe confinement area should be selected. If the dog is trained to a crate or exercise pen, either of these may be used. If the dog is not trained to a crate, and such confinement must be used to prevent destructiveness, elimination, or self-trauma, barrier frustration can result and can lead to self-trauma as the dog attempts to escape. This can lead to an apparent worsening of the condition. This form of restriction should be considered temporary and should be abandoned as soon as possible.

To enhance the dog's well-being and promote positive interactions between the dog and owner, a daily exercise, positive training, and play time should be scheduled.

Behavior Management

Specific behavior management instructions have not been subjected to experimental validation. Specialists agree that retrospective reprimand and physical punishment should be stopped [8,29]. Specific instructions that promote independent interactions between the owner and dog and are provided in phases may be the most efficacious [29]. One study suggested that compliance is improved with five or fewer instructions regarding management, however [17].

To enhance compliance with the behavioral program, in several studies [5,30], behavior management is divided into three phases: when the owner is at home, preparing for departure, and returning home (Table 2). In general, the owner should reward calm obedient behavior and should not reward clingy attention-seeking behavior. Particularly in cases of hyperattachment, reinforcement of social attention seeking may impede independence training that prepares the dog to be alone. If the dog engages in climbing or jumping up on the owner, whining, or nudging, the owner should turn or walk away, not reinforcing the attention-seeking behavior with visual contact, petting, or

Table 2
Behavior management program for separation anxiety

Time	Behavior modification
At home	Do not punish
	Praise calm, obedient behavior
	Encourage "independence," resting without physical contact between the dog and owner
	Practice daily, not associated with departure, positive exercises that teach the dog to lie down and stay in place calmly as the owner moves away; eventually, this forms the basis for graduated departures
	Give departure cues (eg, pick up keys or purse, put on work shoes) at times not associated with departure; ignore dog's active response
Before leaving	Ignore the dog 30 minutes before departure
	Leave calmly in a low-key manner
	Leave a safe treat-filled toy on departure
When returning	Do not punish retrospectively
	Ignore dog until it is calm

Data from Refs. [5,22,29,30].

talking. For special attention at other times, the owner should call the dog to her or him and then give attention when the dog is calm.

Medication

Behavioral medication may play a role in the treatment of separation anxiety. Medication can decrease anxiety and arousal so that a behavior modification plan can be implemented more successfully. When medication is added at the initial phase of treatment in conjunction with a behavioral program, more animals may respond more quickly compared with controls [5,30]. Behavior modification alone [33] or medication alone [34] may be as effective after several months of treatment. Shortening the latency to response may help owners to retain animals in their homes, however.

There is debate about the merits of starting medication at the onset of treatment [22,35] and the effectiveness of medication beyond its potential sedating side effects [29]. Several large multicentric studies compared behavior modification alone (placebo control) with behavior modification plus behavioral medication (treatment), however. Compared with controls, more dogs that received behavior modification plus medication responded more quickly. In general, this difference persisted until, at 4 to 6 weeks, the control groups "caught up" with the treated group. This trend suggests that, given time, behavior modification alone can be as effective as behavior modification combined with behavioral medication. In the authors' experience, however, cases of separation anxiety often do not have much time. By the time consultation by the veterinarian is sought, relinquishment or even euthanasia may be imminent. In addition, separation anxiety is a serious welfare problem because of the distress that dogs experience in states of anxiety or fear. Therefore, starting medication sooner rather than later is often to be recommended on welfare grounds. The goal is to reduce anxiety and fear as quickly as possible so that new conditioned (learned) responses can be established. With time, medication may be withdrawn, although some cases may continue to be managed best with some level of antianxiety medication.

Medication may be used on a daily basis or as needed for anxiety. The former approach may be best for cases of separation anxiety. For specific and predictable phobic behavior associated with isolation, such as thunderstorm phobia, administration of medication before an anxiety-producing event but not at other times may be effective. The third strategy [36] combines daily medication ("baseline") with as needed "adjunctive" medication, such as when storms arise or when two owners are leaving simultaneously, which may have an additive effect on separation anxiety for some dogs.

Two psychotropic medications have been approved by the US Food and Drug Administration for the treatment for canine separation anxiety. Clomipramine (Clomicalm), a tricyclic compound, has been on the market for many years. Fluoxetine (Reconcile), a selective serotonin reuptake inhibitor, was approved in 2007. In a large, double-blind, placebo-controlled, multicentric clinical trial, significantly more dogs given fluoxetine (1–2 mg/kg/d) with behavioral management, compared with placebo with behavioral management, improved (as measured by overall severity score) during all but 1 week of the 8-week trial [5]. Ultimately, 72% of dogs treated with fluoxetine and behavior management improved compared with 50% of placebo (behavior management only) dogs [5]. In a sister study that compared fluoxetine with placebo for 8 weeks without behavior management instructions, improvement was observed in 65% of dogs with separation anxiety that received fluoxetine compared with 51% of dogs that received placebo [34].

In clinical trials, fluoxetine [5] and clomipramine [30] have established efficacy and safety for several months of treatment. In clinical practice, longer treatment durations may be needed. The authors' treatment plan is to continue medication until 2 months after a satisfactory response and then to discontinue gradually if possible. The behavioral management program should continue. Animals that relapse when medication is withdrawn may resume therapy. Clinical experience has proved these drugs to be well tolerated for months to years of treatment. Some dogs may require lifelong treatment at the lowest effective dose. Such dogs should be examined annually and screened with routine laboratory evaluation, including a complete blood cell count, serum chemistry, and urinalysis (if indicated).

Dogs that fail to show a satisfactory response at approved doses may require extra-label medical treatment, higher doses or adjunctive agents. Before such an approach, the possibility of medical differentials should be reconsidered and the behavioral management plan should be reviewed. In multidog households, the possibility that more than one dog exhibits signs of separation anxiety should be ruled out with serial confinement or videotape monitoring.

A second agent may be added as an adjunctive agent to enhance the effect of fluoxetine or clomipramine [36,37]. Adjunctive agents include buspirone, diazepam, alprazolam, lorazepam, or trazodone [37]. Note that to avoid the possibility of serotonin syndrome, a selective serotonin reuptake inhibitor and tricyclic compound should not be used concurrently with a monoamine oxidase inhibitor, such as selegiline. Pheromone treatment (Dog Appeasement Pheromone [DAP]; Ceva Animal Health, Inc., Lenexa, Kansas) may also be used; in one study of dogs with separation-related disorders, pheromone treatment compared favorably with clomipramine treatment [31].

Outcome Measures

Because of the latency, over weeks to months, for satisfactory resolution of signs, it is imperative that owners monitor specific target signs of improvement to recognize treatment success or failure. Specific signs should be identified and rated in a behavioral diary with respect to frequency, intensity, and duration. For example, urinations in the house can be counted daily and noted to monitor progress. Subjective signs, such as destructiveness, can be rated daily on a five-point scale (from 0 = absent to 5 = worst). In this way, the client and clinician can quantify improvement. Adverse events and medication changes can also be noted on the behavioral diary.

The conditions under which the dog displays clinical signs of separation distress are the "eliciting contexts." Clients can often describe these in detail, in terms of day of week, time of day, number of persons departing simultaneously, and so on. The frequency at which clinical signs are detected should be recorded as a function of the number of departures, also called "separation anxiety–related departure" (SARD) [5]. If, for example, the dog exhibits clinical signs when the owner departs in the evenings or on weekends but not for work, the average number of SARDS per week can be calculated (eg, seven), and the number of these that result in separation anxiety signs can be computed (eg, five). The actual percent of SARDs that involved clinical signs can then be calculated (five of seven = approximately 70%) and used as a basis for monitoring progress.

In general, with appropriate treatment, approximately 60% to 80% of cases of separation anxiety show improvement over time [17,33]. In one study, mixed-breed dogs were less likely to improve than purebred dogs [17]. Approximately 15% remain the same, and less than 6% worsen. In contrast, if not treated, 45% of separation anxiety cases improve, whereas 36% worsen [33]. In one study of 52 dogs treated for separation anxiety, 80% were retained but 8% were relinquished and 12% were euthanized (N = 52) [17].

Thunderstorm phobia can compound separation distress, such that dogs that marginally tolerate separation become intolerant when thunderstorms arise and they are alone (class C). A history of separation distress does not predict that thunderstorm phobia is likely to result, however.

There is also an overlap in the diagnosis of separation anxiety and thunderstorm phobia. Clinicians report that during "thunderstorm season," when storms can become a daily occurrence in certain geographic areas of the United States, dogs that experience storm phobia manifest signs of separation anxiety as well. In one study of 51 dogs presented to a university behavior clinic with behavioral signs of anxiety, 49% were diagnosed with separation anxiety alone, 10% were diagnosed with noise or storm phobia alone, and 41% had separation anxiety and storm or noise phobia [38]; thus, it is appropriate to consider these two problems together.

NOISE SENSITIVITY

There are two further reasons to consider aversion to noise alongside separation-related problems. First, there is evidence that the occurrence of either problem affects the likelihood of the occurrence of the other. Second, it is possible for one to be mistaken for the other. For example, elimination in the owner's absence is not necessarily associated with separation-related anxiety but may occur in response to the distress caused by a particular noise stimulus that occurred in the owner's absence, such as a thunderstorm or firework event. Such an event might also predispose an animal previously comfortable when left alone to heightened distress when left alone. Careful investigation is necessary to discern the primary from the secondary problem. Patients that have one problem should therefore be screened for the other as a matter of routine, and cases should be investigated thoroughly to minimize the risk for delayed or inappropriate intervention.

A distress response to noise is often described as a fear or phobia, but these terms are often poorly differentiated in writings on the subject. Their use excludes other responses indicative of suffering that can occur concurrently, such as normal and pathologic anxiety [1,8,39–44]. In this section, the term *noise sensitivity* or *aversion* is used, unless there is specific justification for another term.

Distress responses to sounds take a variety of forms, ranging from more mild reactions, such as panting, hiding, hyperactivity, or escape attempts [43], to more extreme reactions, such as destructiveness and self-trauma. As a result, many owners may seek help and advice from veterinarians, behaviorists, and dog trainers [45] or elect relinquishment, abandonment, or euthanasia [16,45,46]. Between 40% and 50% of dog owners report that their dog is "scared" of some sort of noise [42,47]. It is therefore, without doubt, a major welfare concern.

Sensitivity to noise is among the most common behavior concerns of owners, although it is frequently inadequately or ineffectively treated. Treatment is often delayed until problematic responses are extreme, such as occurs with panic reactions or reactions to multiple stimuli. Animals with these problems may be perfectly normal at other times and may not be described temperamentally as fearful [1]. Although these problems may affect up to half of the dogs in a given area [7], a review of the caseload of the Association of Pet Behavior Counsellors suggested that they made up less than 10% of the reported referrals [48]. Thus, although these problems seem to be common, they do not seem to be commonly referred for specialist treatment. There is enormous potential for their management in general veterinary practice.

When polled, just less than one third of dog owners reported that they would actually seek advice for the treatment of a noise fear, and approximately 15% said that they would seek help from their veterinarian [47]. So, for every 3 cases that are reported in practice, 17 cases may go unmentioned.

Recently, there have been several significant advances in our understanding of noise-related problems through the publication of several carefully monitored clinical trials [49–53] and epidemiologic studies [1,47,54–57]. These studies question the specificity of current regimens and are likely to change the way we investigate these problems. The authors review the conclusions and implications of these studies in the following sections.

History of Onset, Clinical Signs, and Related Factors

In a survey of more than 3500 dog owners recruited on-line, the presentation of signs and the risk factors associated with noise sensitivity were reviewed [56,57]. In this sample, the largest to date, 2577 owners reported having a noise-aversive dog. The most commonly reported noise aversions were to fireworks (n = 836), followed by thunderstorms (n = 817) and gunshots (n = 430). There was an association between the pattern of onset (ie, whether the problem was acute or not or appeared after first exposure) and specific noise fear (Fig. 1). A history of nonacute onset ranged from 23% (37 of 160) among those dogs scared of party poppers to 61% for those scared of thunderstorms (497 of 817). Only for an aversion to thunderstorm noises was the proportion of dogs with nonacute onset greater than 50% [56,57].

A particularly interesting finding is that reported behavioral signs tended to partition more clearly on the basis of the history of onset than on the basis of

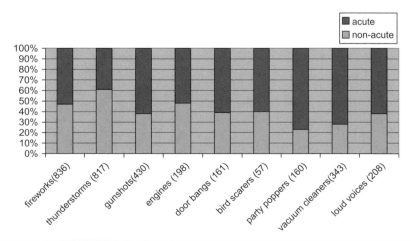

Fig. 1. Onset history (acute versus nonacute or gradual) for the nine most commonly reported noise sensitivities in a population of 3516 dogs. Numbers in brackets refer to the number of dogs affected in each column. The distribution of acute versus nonacute onset across the different stimuli is not even ($P<.001$).

type of noise [56,57]. For example, by owner report, dogs with nonacute onset typically showed signs of panting, pacing, restlessness, hypervigilance, inappetence, trembling, and more frequent elimination. These might be considered signs of autonomic arousal associated with anxiety or anticipation of an impending aversive event. By owner report, however, dogs with a history of acute onset more commonly showed signs, such as hiding, cowering, and "being jumpy," in response to noises. These behaviors suggest an overt fear avoidance strategy. The important conclusion is that acute-onset problems seem to be associated with a fear response; non–acute-onset problems seem to be associated with an anxiety response.

There were also significant associations between these factors and breed, the age the dog was obtained, and the age of the dog at onset of the problem. Hounds, toy breeds, and mixed breeds more commonly reported an acute-onset history with fear-related problems, whereas terriers, entire bitches, and dogs rehomed around 1 month of age more typically reported a nonacute onset [56,57].

It is often assumed that the onset of noise avoidance responses (stimulus aversion) is associated with the trauma of exposure. Data from Iimura and his colleagues [56,57] suggest, however, that this is not the situation in most cases. Other possible mechanisms for the development of stimulus aversion include a lack of habituation, stress-induced dishabituation, sensitization, and social transmission. The role of habituation in the prevention of fears is well documented [58]. Iimura [56] found that exposure to fireworks, engine noises, door bangs, party poppers, vacuum cleaners, and loud voices as a juvenile, younger than 6 months of age, seemed to have a protective effect.

Juvenile exposure to one stimulus, engine noises, seemed particularly important, possibly suggesting that this specific exposure might be a marker of generalized socialization [56,57]. This would be consistent with the finding of Appleby and colleagues [58], who found that dogs not exposed at an early age to an urban environment (which would presumably include exposure to engine noises) were, as adults, more prone to exhibit avoidance behavior and aggressive responses in a wide range of environments. Alternately, it might be that the ability to see a clear stimulus in association with the noise, which approaches as the noise gets louder and fades as it goes away but never does any harm or comes too close, helps the animal to learn that loud noises are not dangerous; however, if they are unable to see anything clearly in association with a noise, such as might occur with thunderstorms or fireworks, it might be that there remains a significant element of uncertainty.

Social transmission is a possible explanation for aversive responses. Iimura [56] found that 22.6% of the 283 owners with more than one noise-sensitive dog claimed that one of their animals had learned or copied another dog's fear. There was no evidence for the social transmission of an aversion to noises from people, which is consistent with the physiologic data of Dreschel and Granger [59].

Sensitization describes the development of an aversion over time not as a result of a specific traumatic episode but attributable to the cumulative effect of repeated stimulus exposure and repeated minor stress responses. Most (61%) dogs with an aversion to thunderstorms seemed to develop this problem over an extended period [56]. Other commonly reported noise sensitivities with a prolonged onset were an aversion to engine noises (48%) and fireworks (47%) [56]. Of the common noise aversions, these stimuli are most likely to occur in bouts or series of loud noises, separated by brief periods of quiet. The pattern of stimulus presentation may be critical to the sensitization process.

Stress-induced dishabituation describes the loss of a specific habituated response as a result of exposure to unrelated stressors. This phenomenon is well documented in people but has not been given much attention in the veterinary behavior literature. Iimura [56] found an association between nonspecific signs of stress (eg, digestive upset, binge eating) and the occurrence of a noise fear, however. Although it is not possible to determine the nature of the relation among these factors, the data did reveal that a proportion of subjects exhibited these nonspecific signs before the onset of the fear. The possible association between stress factors and the development of noise aversion deserves the attention of researchers and clinicians. If stress-induced dishabituation is suspected, management of underlying stress factors must be addressed if the case is to be resolved.

TREATMENT REGIMENS

Recent studies have evaluated the efficacy of several treatment regimens for various noise sensitivities, although study designs did not include placebo controls. These include the use of clomipramine and alprazolam in combination with behavior modification for the control of reactions to thunderstorms [49], the use of DAP in combination with ignoring problematic behavior [50], and the use of DAP within a compact disk (CD)–based training program [51]. Another study casts some doubt on the relative importance of specific recommendations used in these studies. Cracknell and Mills [53] investigated the effect of a homeopathic preparation for the management of an aversion to firework noises against a placebo, in combination with a minimal behavioral therapy regimen (ignoring the dog's responses). The results revealed a significant improvement in both groups; however, there was no evidence that the homeopathic preparation was superior to a placebo. The level of improvement (65% of cases improved, 50% overall reduction in severity of clinical signs, and 72.5% reported owner satisfaction) is comparable to that reported in the other clinical studies, however (Fig. 2). There is clearly a need for further work focusing on the efficacy and detail of specific elements of treatment.

The theory behind the use of sound recordings to desensitize and countercondition animals to noise sensitivity is well established [60], but a recent study by Levine and Mills [52] have examined more closely its implementation in practice. Owners, each with a dog with an aversion to firework noise, were closely monitored over a 12-month period [52]. During this time, owners

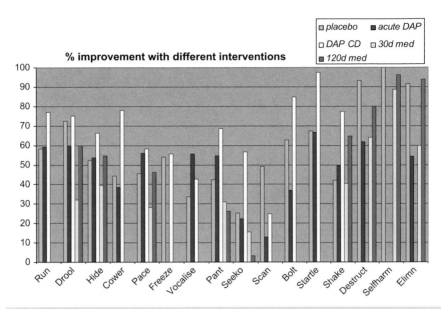

Fig. 2. Reported change in individual signs in response to different interventions. Placebo data are taken from Cracknell and Mills [53], Dog Appeasement Pheromone (DAP) CD data from Levine and colleagues [51], acute DAP data from Mills (unpublished), and 30-day and 120-day medication data from Crowell Davis and colleagues [49].

exposed their dogs to one of two different CD-based training programs in combination with DAP to desensitize their dogs to firework noise. Clients were also advised to create a "safe haven" for their dog (ie, a place to which the animal could retire at will and to which the dog had been specifically trained to have pleasant associations). No behavioral medication was used. With regard to the CDs, the results indicated that the clarity of instructions provided with the recording rather than the quality of the recording itself was critical to successful implementation. With regard to the safe haven, clients had some difficulty with the concept, often erroneously perceiving it as the location where the animal historically ran when frightened. With the recommended behavioral treatment, most improvement (ie, more than a 70% reduction) was seen in the signs of destructiveness, drooling, freezing, bolting, and startling. By contrast, least improvement was seen in owner seeking, panting, and vigilance [52]. The lower level of reduction in owner-seeking behavior may be attributable to the instruction to ignore the dog's behavior, which can actually lead to a transient intensification of the dog's behavior before its improvement.

There were temporal patterns of interest [52]. The improvements seen at the time of exposure during the month of November (a traditional time for fireworks in the United Kingdom) seemed to be maintained until the new year and for 12 months after the initial sessions, with little retraining. Although not statistically significant, after 12 months, there were trends suggesting a potential deterioration of the beneficial behavioral effect and a need for re-establishing conditioned responses [52]. Most owners reported that the program was easy to follow, and 88% said they would repeat the treatment process if they had another animal with a similar problem. Subjectively, the use of pheromone seemed to enhance the training process [52].

In clinical practice, treatment should consist of two elements:

1. Short-term interventions aimed at the immediate management of a problem when the threat is imminent (eg, just before seasonal firework celebrations)
2. Long-term interventions aimed at the resolution of the problem

In the immediate short-term situation, based on the aforementioned studies, specific instructions of what to do and what not to do should be provided to owners (Box 1). Chemotherapeutic intervention using rapidly acting agents, such as benzodiazepines, may be justified on welfare grounds alone. Table 3 lists the commonly used medications and their indications. It should be noted that phenothiazines are not recommended for general treatment of noise aversions. These drugs produce sedation without attenuating the subjective fear response of the animal and may even potentiate the fear response [40].

Pheromone products may also be useful in the management of the immediate crisis (DAP). Pheromone products do not sedate the animal; thus, pets may

---

Box 1: Advice to owners on how to prepare for and respond to reactions of a noise-aversive dog

1. Do not punish the dog when scared; it only confirms that there is something to be afraid of.
2. Do not fuss or try to reassure the dog, because this rewards the behavior the dog is engaging in at the time.
3. Ignore any fearful behavior that occurs for no good reason, or pretend to be particularly happy as you go about your normal routines.
4. Make sure your dog is kept in a safe and secure environment at all times so that it does not bolt and escape if a sudden noise occurs. The use of DAP may be used to provide an emotionally secure environment.
5. Provide the dog with a safe and secure retreat because this helps it to cope, and thus reduces the intensity of the fear response. The dog should be trained to associate this area with many pleasant experiences not associated with fearful responses. The "safe place" should not simply be a bolt-hole used by the animal only when it is scared. When the season begins, it may help to black out one of the quietest rooms in the house and place toys there for your pet to play with and preferably things for you to do as well, such that the room is associated with positive experiences. Blacking out the room removes the potentially additional problems of flashing lights, for example, in the case of firework or thunderstorm fears.

Adapted from Cracknell NR, Mills DS. A double-blind placebo-controlled study into the efficacy of a homeopathic remedy for fear of firework noises in the dog (*Canis familiaris*). Vet J 2008;177:80–8; with permission.

still startle in response to aversive noises, although with pheromone treatment, the animal should recover more quickly. Owners need to be so advised.

In the longer term, the animal's perception of noise must be altered, using sound recordings, by the process of systematic desensitization. First, sounds that resemble but are not identical to the problem stimulus should be played at such a low intensity that the animal does not react inappropriately to the recordings. Gradually, the volume is increased. The program may be speeded up by playing the recordings for short periods frequently rather than for extended periods and by using a DAP pheromone diffuser during training. The next stage involves encouraging a response that is counter to the problem behavior, a process called counterconditioning. This might be a relaxation exercise or play or a formal obedience command, such as "down-stay." Counterconditioning is particularly important for controlling the anxiety component to the problem. Medication, such as a tricyclic antidepressant (TCA) or selective serotonin reuptake inhibitor (SSRI), may be indicated during this process (see Table 3). Benzodiazepines are not recommended during this process because they may inhibit learning. In cases in which the problem is associated with a high level of attention seeking, this behavior must also be addressed by encouraging the pet to be more independent. Clients should expect to see most progress in the first 4 weeks of this process.

Long-term management is necessary for long-term success. Regular follow-up contact should be scheduled. Group classes may motivate change, allow efficient use of resources, and help owners to share their problem with others who are similarly troubled. Annual re-exposure treatment is recommended. This can be managed in practice by sending out reminders to again implement the behavioral training, in much the same way that immunization reminders are sent out each year.

PROGNOSIS

The differentiation of signs described previously has recently prompted a reanalysis of several of the studies involving noise-sensitive dogs, which was conducted at the University of Lincoln by one of the authors (DSM). This suggests that several intervention strategies, including the use of DAP, with minimal behavior therapy [50] and a desensitization program (Daniel S. Mills, unpublished study, 2001) produce more effect on the signs of fear than anxiety, especially in the early stages of treatment. Thus, it might be argued that initial intervention reduces the response to the stimulus when it is present (ie, the fear response) but has less effect on the anticipation of the problem (ie, the anxiety component), which obviously involves a greater element of learning, may not always be associated with the actual occurrence of the unpleasant event, and thus is more resistant to extinction. The clear differentiation of a noise aversion to an anxiety versus a fear-related problem on the basis of the predominant signs would therefore seem to be of clinical treatment and prognostic relevance and deserves attention in future studies.

Table 3
Commonly used behavioral drugs for anxieties, fears, phobias, and aversions of dogs

Drug class	Drug name	Oral dose and frequency	Side effects	Comments	Reference
Phenothiazine	Acepromazine	0.1–2.2 mg/kg PRN for storms, fireworks	Ataxia, relaxation of third eyelid, behavioral disinhibition	Tranquilizer rather than an antianxiety agent May be useful for mild or infrequent fears, not satisfactory for chronic use	[33]
BZ	Diazepam (Valium)	0.5–2.2 mg/kg PRN for storms	May inhibit learning, may release inhibition (including aggression)	Rapid onset of action, rapidly metabolized All BZs may be used with TCAs or SSRIs	[61,62]
BZ	Alprazolam (Xanax)	0.25–3.0 mg/dog PRN for storms 0.02 mg/kg PRN (with clomipramine) 0.01–0.1 mg/kg PRN Maximum of 4 mg/d per dog	Paradoxic excitation Discontinuation reaction (agitation, tremors) if abruptly withdrawn after chronic use To withdraw, reduce dose by 25% per week	Use to help control fearful response to specific events Start dosing 1 hour before fearful event anticipated Use lower dose range if using in combination with clomipramine	[17,49,61]
BZ	Lorazepam (Ativan)	0.02–0.1 mg/kg q 8–24 hours	Side effects are uncommon	Minimally sedating, may require 4 weeks to peak effect	[61]
BZ	Clorazepate (Tranxene)	0.55–2.2 mg/kg q 8–24 hours	Sedation, withdrawal syndrome if chronic use Requires an acid environment for absorption	May be used with TCAs or SSRIs	[17]

Azaperone	Buspirone (Buspar)	1–2 mg/kg q12h	Mild GIT side effects (uncommon), changes in social behavior may be evident	May be used with TCAs or SSRIs	[17,61]
TCA	Amitriptyline (Elavil)	1–3 mg/kg q 12 hours or 2–4 mg q 24 hours	Mild sedation, anticholinergic effects, mild GIT effects	Bitter taste, generally well tolerated, may add BZ	[17,61]
TCA	Clomipramine (Clomicalm)[a]	2–4 mg/kg q 24 hours or 1–3 mg/kg q 12 hours 2 mg/kg q 12 hours	FDA approved for separation anxiety, mild sedation, cardiac conduction disturbances in precisposed patients (human beings)	Use long-term during seasonal noise fears, may add BZ	[9,30,49,61,63]
SSRI	Fluoxetine (Reconcile)[a]	1–2 mg/kg q 24 hours	Mild anticholinergic signs Mild sedation or irritability GIT, especially inappetence Seizures are a contraindication	Use long term during seasonal noise fears, may add BZ	[5]
SSRI	Paroxetine (Paxil)	1 mg/kg q 24 hours	Anticholinergic effects, restlessness		[61,62]
SSRI	Sertraline (Zoloft)		GIT side effects	Start at low dose and titrate up to avoid GIT side effects	[61,62]
SSRI	Citalopram (Celexa)		Cardiac fatalities in beagle dogs at high doses (8 mg/kg/d) in one study	Escitalopram (Lexapro) is an L-isomer	[61,62]

(continued on next page)

Table 3
(continued)

Drug class	Drug name	Oral dose and frequency	Side effects	Comments	Reference
Atypical antidepressant	Trazodone (Desyrel)	2–5 mg/kg PO PRN storms Maximum 300 mg/dose	Sedation GIT side effects, especially with initial doses Paraphimosis is rare side effect in human beings, not noted in canine castrates (BL Sherman, personal observation 1996–2007)	Drug tolerance is common, may need to titrate dose up over time, may be maximum effective dose (estimate 300 mg)	[36,61,62,64] [37]
Beta-blocker	Propranolol	2–3 mg q 12 hours	Generally well tolerated in healthy animals	Use to control autonomic signs May be combined with phenobarbital	[61,62,65]
MAO-B inhibitor	Selegiline	0.5–1 mg/kg q 24 hours in the morning	Do not use with TCAs or SSRIs to avoid serotonin syndrome	Use in cases of inhibited (frozen) fear when the animal does not explore the environment	[61,62]

Note: All drugs administered orally. When using medication, baseline biochemical, hematologic, and electrocardiographic parameters should be established. To increase efficacy in the short and long term, behavioral medication should be used in combination with behavioral management.
When drugs are used as part of a treatment program for behavior problems, the authors suggest that practitioners read the article by Seibert elsewhere in this issue and any listed references. For those drugs that are not licensed for veterinary use, doses, indications, side effects, and contraindications may not be adequately studied and practitioners should be familiar with the published literature and dispense these medications with informed consent.

Abbreviations: BZ, benzodiazepine; FDA, Food and Drug Administration; GIT, gastrointestinal; MAO, monamine oxidase; PRN, as needed; q, every.

[a]FDA approved for treatment of canine separation anxiety in combination with behavioral management.

Other prognostic information has been suggested from the work of Mills and colleagues [54] and Gandia Estelles and colleagues [55]. They report that less success is reported by owners when medication is prescribed, with some evidence to suggest that this might be the result of poorer compliance with the necessary behavior therapy program. They also found that the frequency rather than the duration of exposure to the recording seemed to be a better prognostic indicator, with a more favorable outcome achieved by those who played the recording more frequently. They found that the response to treatment was not predicted from any of the following: the duration of the problem, the number of signs shown, owner rating of severity when using a global scale, or the sum of the frequency times the intensity of the individual signs shown. This suggests that the severity or duration of the problem should not be seen as a deterrent or excuse to intervene. Curiously, a desensitization program seems to be more successful for animals that exhibit fear of fireworks and a fear of thunder compared with animals that have just one of these fears. Perhaps this results from greater owner commitment in these circumstances. Levine and colleagues [51] found that most improvement occurred in the first month; thus, it is particularly important to monitor and encourage owners during this first month. They also found all cases that presented with destructiveness completely resolved this sign.

SUMMARY

As the scientific study of separation anxiety and noise sensitivities grows, so we are gaining a much clearer understanding of the subtleties of the problem. This brings a greater ability to prescribe effective treatment programs accurately and predict their outcome. A correct diagnosis is obviously essential, but careful attention to presenting signs is also warranted, because it seems that a greater response to signs of fear (as opposed to anxiety) is achieved initially in many cases, and owners should be advised accordingly. Owners should be encouraged that it is never too late or a case is never too bad to contemplate treatment, because these factors do not seem to affect prognosis and treatment is relatively straightforward for most owners.

Anxieties, fears, and phobias are common and problematic behavioral complaints of dog owners. This article focuses on the diagnosis and treatment of two such conditions: separation anxiety and noise aversions. Veterinarians are encouraged to recognize and treat such conditions on first presentation to address welfare issues and optimize successful management. New data suggest new treatment modalities. Failure to treat can result in disruption of the human-animal bond and subsequent abandonment, relinquishment, or even euthanasia of the affected dog.

References

[1] McCobb EC, Brown EA, Damiani K, et al. Thunderstorm phobia in dogs: an internet survey of 69 cases. J Am Anim Hosp Assoc 2001;37(4):319–24.
[2] Borchelt PL, Voith VL. Diagnosis and treatment of separation-related behavior problems in dogs. Vet Clin North Am Small Anim Pract 1982;12:625–35.

[3] McCrave EA. Diagnostic criteria for separation anxiety in the dog. Vet Clin North Am Small Anim Pract 1991;21:247–55.

[4] Sherman BL. Separation anxiety in dogs. The Compendium on Continuing Education for the Practicing Veterinarian 2008;30(1):27–42.

[5] Simpson B, Landsberg GM, Reisner IR, et al. Effects of Reconcile (Fluoxetine) chewable tablets plus behavior management for canine separation anxiety. Vet Ther 2007;8(1):18–31.

[6] Guthrie A. Dogs behaving badly—canine separation disorder research. Veterinary Practice 1999;31:12–3.

[7] Bradshaw JWS, McPherson JA, Casey RA, et al. Aetiology of separation-related behaviour in domestic dogs. Vet Rec 2002;151:43–6.

[8] Voith VL, Borchelt PL. Separation anxiety in dogs. In: Voith VL, Borchelt PL, editors. Readings in companion animal behavior. Trenton (NJ): Veterinary Learning Systems; 1996. p. 124–39.

[9] Horwitz DF. Diagnosis and treatment of canine separation anxiety and the use of clomipramine hydrochloride (Clomicalm). J Am Anim Hosp Assoc 2000;37:313–8.

[10] Wright JC, Nesselrote MS. Classification of behavior problems in dogs: distributions of age, breed, sex, and reproductive status. Appl Anim Behav Sci 1987;19:169–78.

[11] Lindell EM. Diagnosis and treatment of destructive behavior in dogs. Vet Clin North Am Small Anim Pract 1997;27(3):533–48.

[12] Patronek GJ, Glickman LT, Back AM, et al. Risk factors for relinquishment of dogs to an animal shelter. J Am Vet Med Assoc 1996;209(4):738–42.

[13] Salman MD, Hutchison J, Ruch-Gallie R. Behavioral reasons for relinquishment of dogs and cats to 12 shelters. J Appl Anim Welf Sci 2000;3:93–106.

[14] Scarlett JM, Salman MD, New JG, et al. The role of veterinary practitioners in reducing dog and cat relinquishments and euthanasias. J Am Vet Med Assoc 2002;220(3): 306–11.

[15] Miller DD, Staats SR, Partlo C, et al. Factors associated with the decision to surrender a pet to an animal shelter. J Am Vet Med Assoc 1996;29(4):738–42.

[16] Segurson SA, Serpell JA, Hart BJ. Evaluation of a behavioral assessment questionnaire for use in the characterization of behavioral problems of dogs relinquished to animal shelters. J Am Vet Med Assoc 2005;227:1755–61.

[17] Takeuchi Y, Houpt KA, Scarlett JM. Evaluation of treatments for separation anxiety. J Am Vet Med Assoc 2000;217:342–5.

[18] Houpt KA, Reisner IR. Breaking the human-companion animal bond. J Am Vet Med Assoc 1996;208:1653–9.

[19] Serpell J, Jagoe JA. Early experience and the development of behavior. In: Serpell JA, editor. The domestic dog: its evolution, behavior, and interactions with people. New York: Cambridge University Press; 1996. p. 79–102.

[20] Flannigan G, Dodman NH. Risk factors and behaviors associated with separation anxiety in dogs. J Am Vet Med Assoc 2001;219(4):460–6.

[21] Perry G, Seksel K, Beer L, et al. Separation anxiety: a summary of some of the characteristics of 61 cases seen at Sydney, Australia, behaviour practice. In: Mills D, Levine E, Landsberg GM, et al, editors. Current issues and research in veterinary behavioral medicine. West Lafayette (IN): Purdue University Press; 2005. p. 203–6.

[22] Appleby D, Pluijmakers J. Separation anxiety in dogs: the function of homeostasis in its development and treatment. Vet Clin North Am Small Anim Pract 2003;33(2):321–44.

[23] Pageat P. Pathologie du comportement du Chien, Du Point Veterinaire. Maisons Alfort (France): 1995.

[24] Voith VL, Wright JC, Danneman PJ. Is there a relationship between canine behavior problems and spoiling activities, anthropomorphism, and obedience training? Appl Anim Behav Sci 1992;34:263–72.

[25] Clark GI, Boyer WN. The effects of dog obedience training and behavioural counseling upon the human-canine relationship. Appl Anim Behav Sci 1993;37:147–59.

[26] Jagoe A, Serpell J. Owner characteristics and interactions and the prevalence of canine behaviour problems. Appl Anim Behav Sci 1996;47:31–44.
[27] Tuber DS, Hennessy MB, Sanders S, et al. Behavioral and glucocorticoid responses of adult dogs (*Canis familiaris*): companionship and social separation. J Comp Psychol 1996;110: 103–8.
[28] Overall KL. Separation anxiety: not all dogs crated or kenneled successfully. DVM Newsmagazine 2003;34:20S–2S.
[29] Podberscek AL, Hsu Y, Serpell JA. Evaluation of clomipramine as an adjunct to behavioural therapy in the treatment of separation-related problems in dogs. Vet Rec 1999;145:365–9.
[30] King JN, Simpson BS, Overall KL, et al. Treatment of separation anxiety in dogs with clomipramine: results from a prospective, randomized, double-blind, placebo-controlled, parallel-group, multicenter clinical trial. Appl Anim Behav Sci 2000;67:255–75.
[31] Gaultier E, Bonnafous L, Bougrat L, et al. Comparison of the efficacy of a synthetic dog-appeasing pheromone with clomipramine for the treatment of separation-related disorders in dogs. Vet Rec 2005;156:533–8.
[32] Lund JD, Jorgensen MC. Behaviour patterns and time course of activity in dogs with separation problems. Appl Anim Behav Sci 1999;63:219–36.
[33] Voith VL, Ganster D. Separation anxiety: review of 42 cases. Proceedings of the American Veterinary Medical Association Annual Meeting, Boston, 1992.
[34] Landsberg GM, Melese P, Sherman BL. Effectiveness of fluoxetine chewable tablets in the treatment of canine separation anxiety. Journal of Veterinary Behavior, Clinical Applications and Research 2008;3(1):12–9.
[35] Casey RA. Use of clomipramine for separation anxiety in dogs. Vet Rec 1998;142:587–8.
[36] Simpson BS. Behavioral drugs: "baseline" and "adjunctive" agents. Proceedings of the American Veterinary Medical Association 140th Annual Convention, July 15–19, 2006, Honolulu, Hawaii, Session Note #02225, 2006.
[37] Gruen ME, Sherman BL. Use of trazodone as an adjunctive agent in the treatment of canine anxiety disorders: 56 cases (1995–2007). Journal of the American Veterinary Medical Association 2008; in press.
[38] Overall KL, Dunham AE, Frank D. Frequency of nonspecific clinical signs in dogs with separation anxiety, thunderstorm phobia, and noise phobia, alone or in combination. J Am Vet Med Assoc 2001;219(4):467–73.
[39] Landsberg GM, Hunthausen W, Ackerman L. Handbook of behavior problems of the dog and cat. 2nd edition. Philadephia: Saunders/Elsevier Health Sciences; 2003.
[40] Overall KL. Clinical behavioral medicine for small animals. St. Louis (MO): Mosby; 1996. p. 209–50.
[41] Tuber DS, Hothersall D, Peters MF. Treatment of fears and phobias in dogs. Vet Clin North Am Small Anim Pract 1982;12(4):607–23.
[42] Beaver BV. Canine behavior: a guide for veterinarians. Philadelphia: WB Saunders; 1999.
[43] Shull-Selcer EA, Stagg W. Advances in the understanding and treatment of noise phobias. Vet Clin North Am Small Anim Pract 1991;21(2):353–68.
[44] Askew HR. Treatment of behavior problems in dogs and cats: a guide for the small animal veterinarian. 2nd edition. Oxford (UK): Blackwell Publishing; 2003.
[45] Rugbjerg H, Proschowsky HF, Ersboll AK, et al. Risk factors associated with interdog aggression and shooting phobias among purebred dogs in Denmark. Prev Vet Med 2003;58: 85–100.
[46] Wells DL, Hepper PG. Prevalence of behaviour problems reported by owners of dogs purchased from an animal rescue shelter. Appl Anim Behav Sci 2000;69:55–65.
[47] Blackwell E, Casey R, Bradshaw J. Firework fears and phobias in the domestic dog. 2005. Reports prepared for the RSPCA. Available at: http://www.rspca.org.uk/servlet/ Satellite?blobcol=urlblob&blobheader=application%2Fpdf&blobkey=id&blobtable= RSPCABlob&blobwhere=1131368232338&ssbinary=true. Accessed June 12, 2008.

[48] Association of Pet Behaviour Counsellors (APBC). Annual review of cases 2005. Available at: http://www.apbc.org.uk/resources/review_2005.pdf. Accessed June 12, 2008.

[49] Crowell-Davis SL, Seibert LM, Sung W, et al. Use of clomipramine, alprazolam, and behavior modification for treatment of storm phobic dogs and their caregivers. J Am Vet Med Assoc 2003;226:744–8.

[50] Sheppard G, Mills DS. Evaluation of dog appeasing pheromone as a potential treatment for dogs fearful of fireworks. Vet Rec 2003;152:432–6.

[51] Levine ED, Ramos D, Mills DS. A prospective study of two self help CD based desensitization and counter-conditioning programmes with the use of Dog Appeasing Pheromone for the treatment of firework fears in dogs. Appl Anim Behav Sci 2007;105:311–29.

[52] Levine ED, Mills DS. Long term follow-up of the efficacy of a behavioural treatment programme for dogs with firework fears. Vet Rec 2008;162:657–9.

[53] Cracknell NR, Mills DS. A double-blind placebo-controlled study into the efficacy of a homeopathic remedy for fear of firework noises in the dog (Canis familiaris). Vet J 2008;177:80–8.

[54] Mills DS, Estelles MG, Coleshaw PH, et al. Retrospective analysis of the treatment of firework fears in dogs. Vet Rec 2003;153:561–2.

[55] Gandia Estelles M, Mills DS, Coleshaw PH, et al. A retrospective analysis of relationships with severity of signs of fear of fireworks and treatment outcome in 99 cases. In: Mills D, Levine E, Landsberg G, et al, editors. Current issues and research in veterinary behavioural medicine—papers presented at the 5th International Veterinary Behavior Meeting. West Lafayette (IN): Purdue University Press; 2005. p. 161–4.

[56] Iimura K. The nature of noise fear in domestic dogs [MPhil thesis]. University of Lincoln, 2006.

[57] Iimura K, Mills DS, Levine E. An analysis of the relationship between the history of development of sensitivity to loud noises and behavioural signs in domestic dogs. In: Landsberg G, Mattiello S, Mills D, editors. Proceedings of the 6th International Veterinary Behaviour Meeting and European College of Veterinary Behavioural Medicine—Companion Animals and European Society of Veterinary Clinical Ethology, Fondazionne Iniziative Zooprofilattiche e Zootechniche, Brescia 2007;70–71.

[58] Appleby DL, Bradshaw JWS, Casey RA. Relationship between aggressive and avoidance behaviour by dogs and their experience in the first six months of life. Vet Rec 2002;150:434–8.

[59] Dreschel N, Granger G. Physiological and behavioral reactivity to stress in thunderstorm-phobic dogs and their caregivers. Appl Anim Behav Sci 2005;95:153–68.

[60] Hothersall D, Tuber DS. Fears in companion dogs: characteristics and treatment. In: Keehn JD, editor. Psychopathology in animals. New York: Academic Press; 1979. p. 239–55.

[61] Simpson BS, Papich MG. Pharmacologic management in veterinary behavioral medicine. Vet Clin North Am Small Anim Pract 2003;33:365–9.

[62] Mills DS, Simpson BS. Psychotropic agents. In: Horwitz D, Mills D, Heath S, editors. BSAVA manual of canine and feline behavioural medicine. Gloucester (UK): British Small Animal Veterinary Association; 2002. p. 237–48.

[63] Hewson CJ. Clomipramine and behavioural therapy in the treatment of separation-related problems in dogs. Vet Rec 2000;146:111–2.

[64] King JN, Overall KL, Appleby D, et al. Results of a follow-up investigation to a clinical trial testing the efficacy of clomipramine in the treatment of separation anxiety in dogs. Appl Anim Behav Sci 2004;89:233–42.

[65] Walker R, Fisher J, Neville P. The treatment of phobias in the dog. Appl Anim Behav Sci 1997;52:275–89.

Vet Clin Small Anim 38 (2008) 1107–1130

VETERINARY CLINICS
SMALL ANIMAL PRACTICE

Canine Aggression Toward Familiar People: A New Look at an Old Problem

Andrew U. Luescher, DVM, PhD[a],*,
Ilana R. Reisner, DVM, PhD[b]

[a]Animal Behavior Clinic, Department of Veterinary Medicine, Purdue University School of Veterinary Medicine, Veterinary Clinical Sciences, LYNN 625 Harrison Street, West Lafayette, IN 47907-2026, USA
[b]Department of Clinical Studies–Philadelphia, School of Veterinary Medicine, University of Pennsylvania, 3900 Delancey Street, Philadelphia, PA 19104-6010, USA

A ggression, and specifically aggression toward owners, is the behavior problem most often referred to behavior specialists (Appendix 1) [1]. Although this complaint is common, it also is frequently misunderstood. In this article, the authors question the traditional explanation of owner-directed aggression as related to a dominance–submissiveness relationship between owner and dog, based on research findings, and provide alternative concepts.

To understand canine aggression better, it is necessary to examine canine social behavior and communication.

DOMESTICATION AND CANINE BEHAVIOR

Although dogs and wolves have phylogenetic similarities, they also are quite different. Dogs have been domesticated for at least 12,000 years and have been selected to remain behaviorally immature compared with wolves [2]. This retardation of development, or neoteny, accounts for many of the pronounced behavioral differences between dogs and wolves. Even in adulthood, dogs show many behaviors typical of juvenile wolves: they remain playful, enjoy physical contact, are highly social, and bark, paw, and nuzzle. Some breeds are more highly neotenized and show more of the behaviors characteristic of wolf puppies than other breeds do [3].

Another notable difference between dogs and wolves is that, unlike wolves, feral or free-ranging dogs do not form well-structured packs. Instead, they live in loosely knit groups, typically of two to five unrelated individuals, formed and increased in size by the abandonment or escape of pets [4].

These findings suggest that the extrapolation of wolf social behavior to dogs—or to dogs and their human families— probably is inappropriate.

*Corresponding author. E-mail address: luescher@purdue.edu (A.U. Luescher).

0195-5616/08/$ – see front matter
doi:10.1016/j.cvsm.2008.04.008

BODY LANGUAGE AND CONFLICT BEHAVIORS

Understanding canine communication and body language and in particular understanding conflict behavior allows the veterinarian to draw conclusions regarding a dog's motivation to be aggressive. This understanding also helps predict incidents of aggression and, it is hoped, to avoid experiencing its consequences.

Dogs communicate by using visual, auditory, and olfactory cues [5]. For humans, the visual cues usually are the most obvious, and the olfactory cues are the least salient.

Visual Communication

Depending on the situation, temperament, genetics, and experience of the individual dog, any of the following behaviors and body postures may be displayed in social situations:

- Self-confident and assertive dogs typically carry their body weight forward, with pricked or erect ears and elevated tail.
- Submissive dogs or dogs showing appeasement behavior typically carry their body weight low to the ground and shifted backward, with ears and tail low and close to the body.
- An offensively (rather than defensively) aggressive dog stands tall with ears and tail up and curls the lips with the corner of the mouth forward and only the incisors and canine teeth exposed.
- A direct eye stare indicates a confident dog and may precede offensive aggression. Avoiding eye contact usually indicates some degree of fear, anxiety, or conflict and may be an appeasement behavior.
- Defensively aggressive dogs lower themselves and shift their body weight backward, raise the lips with the corner of the mouth drawn backward, and expose the teeth on the side of the mouth as well as the incisors and canines.
- When a subordinate social partner greets a more dominant one, it shows appeasement behavior with the body lowered and the tail low and wagging very quickly. This behavior is accompanied by muzzle licking and nuzzling, as during food solicitation from a puppy to an adult. It is important to realize that these behaviors are appeasement behaviors and can be shown to any threatening individual, not just toward dominant members of a hierarchy.
- Exaggerated forms of appeasement include rolling over, exposing the belly and urinating
- Piloerection (raised hackles) indicates fear and anxiety.
- Mounting usually is not related to dominance but rather is a conflict behavior indicating some uncertainty related to the other dog (or person).

Conflict Behavior

Dogs often display signals that seem to be contradictory. In addition, they may exhibit behaviors that apparently are out of context, unrelated to those described in the previous section. Such behaviors may be conflict behaviors resulting from stress, frustration, or motivational conflict. Among other reasons, stress frequently results from an environment that is unpredictable and does not give the dog any control over events, such as pleasant or aversive stimuli. Frustration results from the dog's being motivated to perform a behavior but thwarted from performing it. A dog is in motivational conflict if it experiences two opposing motivations, such as for approach and for withdrawal. For example, a dog that wants to socialize with a person but at the same time is afraid of how the person might react is in an approach–withdrawal conflict.

Conflict behaviors include yawning, lip- or muzzle-licking, looking away or toward the ceiling, visually scanning the surroundings, squinting the eyes, licking objects, scratching self, vocalization, and many others. Even aggression may be performed as a conflict behavior. Some conflict behaviors have become part of the normal behavior repertoire of dogs and a means of communication. These behaviors include averting the gaze when a threatening or dominant dog approaches, cowering and tucking the tail, rolling over and possibly urinating, growling and displaying the "submissive grin," and whining. These behaviors have become appeasement behaviors and are used by a low-ranking or fearful dog to inhibit aggression from a dominant dog or a frightening human. The play bow probably is another ritualized conflict behavior. It is a combination of moving forward and an intention movement to jump backward. It has become a means of signaling a nonthreatening approach.

Mounting, which often is interpreted as a sexual behavior, most commonly indicates that the dog experiences a conflict related to the mounted individual.

It is important to keep three things in mind regarding conflict behaviors in the dog. First, any of these behaviors also may be shown when the dog is not in conflict; for example the dog may yawn because it is tired or scratch because it itches. Thus, context always is important when interpreting these behaviors. Second, although ritualized conflict behaviors have become normal or species-typical social behaviors, they also are shown when the dog is in conflict. They therefore do not necessarily indicate that the relationship of owner and dog and is one of dominance and submission, nor do they necessarily allow any interpretation of the relative social position of the dog and owner. Third, it is important to be aware of and observe conflict behaviors, especially in aggressive dogs, because they indicate some degree of stress and uncertainty. Most important, such behaviors may predict imminent aggression and may point toward the reason for aggression. During human–dog interactions and in training, they may indicate that the dog is confused about what is expected or is afraid of the training situation (eg, of punishment-based training). During behavior modification such as systematic desensitization, conflict behaviors may indicate that the training has moved a bit too quickly. If a dog shows conflict behaviors when approached by a person, they indicate that the dog is uncomfortable or fearful relative to that person and may not necessarily indicate anything about social status. Conflict behaviors also should be monitored throughout the treatment of aggression, because they are a more sensitive indicator of stress or conflict than is overt aggression. In fact, close monitoring of conflict behaviors may help avoid overt aggressive responses.

Because conflict behaviors are an indication of underlying stress, punishment (which increases stress) is contraindicated. Even though punishment could be effective in suppressing particular conflict behaviors at the moment, it does not address the cause of the problem and in many cases increases the stress and conflict that lie at the root of the problem. Thus, because punishment does not address the underlying emotional state of the animal, it is likely to increase the conflict behaviors or may eliminate one behavior but induce another conflict behavior. For example, a German Shepherd dog was aggressive (because of motivational conflict) toward its owners when young. The owners were instructed by their trainer to leave a short line on the choke chain and to give a severe choke chain correction to punish the aggression. This technique suppressed the aggression (it "worked" according to the owner). A few days later the dog started tail chasing. It was presented to the behavior clinic for persistent tail chasing (several hours a day) when it was almost 1 year old. In this case, the outward aggressive responses were suppressed, but the underlying emotional state of conflict remained and resulted in the performance of a displacement behavior (ie, tail chasing).

CANINE AGGRESSION
Aggression is not a diagnosis. To approach a problem of canine aggression clinically, a diagnosis must be made first.

Types of Canine Aggression Toward Humans
The following list is a useful clinical classification of canine aggression exhibited toward humans:

1. Fear-induced aggression
2. Resource guarding (possessive aggression)
3. Conflict-related aggression ("dominance aggression")
4. Territorial aggression (toward strangers and unfamiliar dogs)
5. Predatory aggression
6. Play-related aggression
7. Excitement-induced aggression
8. Pain-induced aggression
9. Maternal aggression
10. Disease-induced aggression/Irritable aggression

Most types of aggression also can be redirected toward another person or animal rather than toward the intended target ("redirected aggression") and also often have a learned component.

Neurophysiology and Pharmacology of Aggression
Although play-related aggression directed toward the owner (especially if there is no bite inhibition) and occasionally predatory behavior, which may be directed toward children running or riding on bicycles, can be a problem, these behaviors are considered "nonaffective" or nonemotional behaviors rather

than examples of aggression. This article is concerned primarily with affective aggression.

Although behaviorists discriminate among many different types of aggression according to trigger, target, motivation, and other factors, neurophysiologists discriminate between only two or possibly among three types of aggression. Affective aggression also could be called "social aggression," can be offensive (self-confident) or defensive (fearful), and is associated with a high level of sympathetic arousal. Affective aggression serves to increase the distance between the subject and a threat or nuisance. In contrast, predatory aggression is part of feeding behavior and really should not be called aggression at all. It is regulated by the appetite-regulating centers in the hypothalamus. It does not involve sympathetic arousal, and stimulation of the amygdala inhibits predatory behavior. Play-related aggression may be distinct from the two other types but has not been studied well.

Aggressive responses are preprogrammed in the brain stem, specifically in the periaqueductal gray matter of the midbrain. The expression of offensive aggression is controlled by the hypothalamus and the limbic system, especially the amygdala. The activity of the limbic system is influenced by perception of the environment (sensory systems, including the vomeronasal organ which perceives pheromones) and previous learning processes. In humans, amygdalectomy was recommended for treatment of aggression. The amygdala also is involved in all other emotional responses, however, so amygdalectomy blunts all emotions.

Defensive aggression is controlled by neurons in the periaqueductal gray matter (with input from the amygdala and the hypothalamus). The same centers control flight and immobility, as well as the killing bite, but not stalking and chasing. The hypothalamus and the amygdala are involved in defensive aggression as well by modulating these responses. Amygdalectomy can "tame" wild animals by eliminating fear aggression.

Serotonin is a neurotransmitter that has been implicated in affective aggression. It has been shown that some aggressive dogs have lower serotonin metabolites in the cerebrospinal fluid (CSF) and thus presumably have lower levels of serotonin in the brain [6]. In laboratory animals, destruction of serotonergic neurons increased offensive aggression, whereas increased serotonergic activity at synapses decreased offensive aggression. Injection of serotonergic agonists (serotonin-like substances) into the amygdala decreased aggression. (Interestingly, serotonin agonists, while decreasing aggressiveness, increased social status; serotonin antagonists decreased it.) This finding suggests that serotonin re-uptake inhibitors that reduce the breakdown of serotonin should be useful in treating affective aggression in dogs. For a review of the physiology of aggression, see [7].

Serotonin also is a neurohormone acting at targets that are remote from the site of release (as opposed to a neurotransmitter, which acts locally on receptors in the synapse into which it was released). As a neurohormone, serotonin is believed to have modulatory effects on other neurotransmitter systems such as the dopaminergic system, which also has been implicated in aggression. The neurohormonal role of serotonin in aggression has not been elucidated.

Serotonin reuptake inhibitors are used frequently in the pharmacologic treatment of canine aggression, although conclusive clinical trials are lacking [8,9]. Not every case of owner-directed aggression is an indication for pharmacologic treatment, however, nor is fluoxetine the only or best choice in each case. The indication for a drug and the choice of drug needs to be determined individually, and blood tests assessing liver and kidney function always are indicated before a drug is used.

If fear and anxiety historically have prevented a dog from attacking its target, anxiolytic drugs (particularly benzodiazepines) sometimes can reduce fear and anxiety and thus disinhibit aggression or can have a paradoxical effect and increase anxiety and aggression. Therefore, when drugs are used to treat aggression in dogs, safety and preventive counseling is important, and clinicians should request that the owners sign a liability waiver attesting that they understand that risk. In some cases a muzzle may be used as an additional safety tool.

It also has been reported that tryptophan supplementation of a low-protein diet was successful in diminishing signs of owner-directed aggression [10]. Tryptophan is a precursor of serotonin, and a low-protein diet facilitates its uptake into the brain.

Genetic Basis for Aggression

Genes, of course, do not code for behavior. Rather, they code for proteins that are used as building blocks for the structure of the central nervous system, for enzymes, for neurotransmitters and neurotransmitter receptors, for neurohormones, and for sensory and effector organs, among others. They also affect mRNA folding, if and when other genes are expressed, transcription factors, and secondary messenger systems. Through these more indirect ways, genes do influence the functionality of the central nervous system, motivation, motor patterns, perception of stimuli, and responses to environmental and social stimuli.

A genetic effect on behavior can be demonstrated for qualitative traits by comparing related species or different breeds within the same environment, through the study of twins in different environments, by pedigree analysis, and by producing hybrid crosses. Quantitative effects can be studied through selection and inbreeding experiments. As a consequence of the separation of the gene pools for purebred dogs and some degree of inbreeding, it can be expected that behavior and temperament and the prevalence of behavioral disorders would differ among breeds of dogs. In their classical study, Scott and Fuller [11] found distinct behavioral differences between the breeds that they studied. Emotional responses to test situations varied particularly strongly among breeds. The investigators also found great within-breed variation and suggested that selection for temperament within a given breed should yield results rapidly. Later, Cattell and colleagues [12] tested 101 dogs belonging to five breeds for 15 different behavioral variables and were able to assign the dogs to their breed correctly based on the behavioral measurements. Other studies have revealed breed differences in receptors for dopamine, a neurotransmitter that is involved in emotional and aggressive responses [13–15]. It therefore is not surprising that behavior traits such as excitability and general activity, aggressiveness, reactivity, playfulness, destructiveness, and ease of housetraining differ among breeds [16,17].

Of more interest to breeders are within-breed genetic differences in behavior. Svartberg [18,19] and Svartberg and Forkman [20] identified four personality traits in dogs (ie, aggressiveness, playfulness, curiosity/fearlessness, and chase proneness), the latter three traits forming the super trait, shyness/boldness. Heritability of these traits has been shown to be moderate (29%–40%) for aggressiveness and high (54%–74%) for shyness/boldness [21].

A recent study [22] in Golden Retrievers showed high (80%) heritability of aggressiveness, with only one or few genes determining whether a dog was categorized as aggressive. In Cocker Spaniels, a genetic effect on aggression has been demonstrated by showing that different coat colors are associated with different levels of aggressiveness [23]. In English Springer Spaniels, aggressiveness is associated with a particular sire [24].

These studies show that there is a genetic basis for aggressiveness, that breeds differ in how likely they are to be aggressive, and that selection against aggressiveness should produce rapid results. There currently is no reliable test to measure aggressiveness, however. The best data might rely upon honest reports from dog owners about aggressiveness in real-life situations [19]. It should be noted, however, that the heritability of aggressiveness was found to be only moderate. Therefore, although there is an obvious genetic contribution to a dog's level of aggressiveness, the environment also plays an important role.

CANINE AGGRESSION TOWARD OWNERS
Conflict-related Aggression
Prevalence

Aggression toward owners traditionally was diagnosed most commonly as dominance-related aggression. By definition, dominance-related aggression is directed toward household members in situations in which the social position of the (dominant) dog is challenged.

A recent study at the Atlantic Veterinary College found that 40% of dogs growled at a household member in some situation. More than 20% had growled or snapped over food or objects, and more than 15% bit a household member. About 12% of dogs bit their owners hard enough to leave a mark [25,26].

A survey study of English Springer Spaniels performed at Cornell University [24] showed that more than one fourth of the dogs (26.3%) had a history of biting someone, and about two thirds of these (65.2%) bit familiar people. Approximately, one sixth of the studied population of English Springer Spaniels had bitten a familiar person.

Differential diagnosis

"Aggression toward owners" is neither a diagnosis nor a homogeneous condition: it is likely to have a variety of causes. In a study of CSF neurotransmitter metabolites in aggressive and nonaggressive dogs, only some dogs that were aggressive toward their owners had changes in neurotransmitter levels [6]. In another study, aggressive behavior worsened in some females but not in others after neutering [27]. Some dogs growl before biting, but others do not. Body language is quite variable among affected dogs. Individual affected dogs respond differently to treatment.

Aggression toward household members can have many reasons. Differential diagnoses include "dominance aggression," conflict-related aggression, resource-guarding or possessive aggression (often considered a subtype of conflict-related aggression), fear-induced aggression, play aggression, excitement-induced aggression, and maternal aggression. It should be kept in mind that a dog that is excitable for any reason is more likely to be aggressive (or to show any other behavior problem). Hyperexcitability therefore should be addressed if present.

In cases of canine aggression, it is advisable to perform a physical examination with a basic neurologic examination (which frequently is difficult or impossible because of the aggression), a complete blood cell count, serum chemistry panel, and urinalysis. Medical differentials that should be considered are hepatic encephalopathy, hypothyroidism, and neurologic disorders such as seizures, storage disease, inflammatory and infectious diseases, and brain tumors. It should also be kept in mind that any disease process that makes the dog feel uncomfortable or painful may increase aggression. Such conditions include arthritis, otitis, dermatologic conditions, and any systemic disease. Other conditions that have been mentioned as differentials for aggression include acute renal failure, hypoglycemia, sensory deficits, hydrocephalus, meningoencephalitis, rabies, pseudopregnancy, Cushing's disease, and hypocalcemia [28]. Therefore a veterinarian always should be involved in the clinical treatment of canine aggression.

Diagnosis

The behavior diagnosis is based primarily on historical information regarding the dog's development, its current and past living situation, its temperament, the current presentation, and the development of the behavior disorder, along with a detailed history of recent aggressive incidents. Consequently, the history is broken down into three parts. One contains questions on general pet history and management. The second part addresses temperament by asking the owner to describe the behavior of the pet in a number of every-day situations (eg, its reaction when meeting a stranger on or off the property, when meeting children, when handled or restrained, around the food bowl, and in other situations). The clinician then categorizes the behavior (eg, as fearful behavior, offensive and defensive aggression, excitability). The third part contains information about the actual behavior problem. This information includes general information: when and where the behavior occurs; what triggers the behavior; what behavior is shown (including body language and facial expression); who/what is the target; how people react and how the animal behaves right after an incident; the frequency and severity of the problem; and ways the owner has tried to treat the problem. For the aggression to be diagnosed correctly in individual cases, however, the history must include more than just the nature of the problem at presentation. It needs to consider the early history of the patient, when and how the problem presented initially, and how the problem presents now. Detailed descriptions of incidents are required. It is useful to have clients describe the most recent three and the very first two or three incidents. The description includes the location, the people and dogs present, their behavior just before the aggression, the aggressive behavior including the dog's body language, and the behavior of the dog(s) and people after the aggression. Owner–dog interaction is evaluated, among other things, by asking for descriptions of the owner's reaction to the aggression, of how the owner trains and disciplines the dog, and of the general management of the dog.

Clients are asked to bring along a videotape of the behavior, if possible. In cases of aggression, of course they are not asked to record a biting incident. It is helpful, however, to see how the owner and pet interact with each other in various contexts and what the pet's body language is during these interactions. Clients also are asked to bring along all training tools that they use or have used with their dog and the pet's favorite treats.

Factors associated with owner-directed aggression
As already mentioned, most cases of aggression toward household members have been diagnosed, by convention, as "dominance-related aggression." "Dominance-related aggression" usually is described as aggression toward household members in situations in which the social position of the (dominant) dog is challenged. Often the owners report that the aggression is unprovoked (which only rarely holds true) and may occur without warning. If they can describe the body language, it is often ambivalent between offensive and defensive. Typically, the dog slinks away and "seems remorseful" (ie, shows appeasement behaviors) after the incident.

Consistent with a diagnosis of dominance-related aggression, it often was contended that aggression toward owners is a problem seen typically in intact male dogs about 2 to 3 years of age. It was assumed that the human family replaced the dog's pack, and that these dogs try to gain the top or alpha position. Once they have achieved that goal and are the dominant member of their family pack, they discipline other "pack" members (family) if these challenged the pack leader (the dog). In most cases, however, findings in the history and in the description of the dog's behavior are inconsistent with this traditional understanding of aggression directed toward household members. In fact, a careful analysis of clinical cases and newer research findings, as well as theoretic considerations, put the validity of a diagnosis of "dominance-related aggression" into question. The following sections present some more recent findings on aggression to household members.

Genetics
The study performed at the Atlantic Veterinary College found English Springer Spaniels and miniature breeds to be overrepresented among the biting dogs [26]. The Cornell survey of English Springer Spaniels owners reported that show dogs, being bred by a "hobby breeder," (choices for source in the survey included "hobby breeder/private home," "professional breeder/kennel," self, previous owner, pet store, and shelter), and being bred at one particular kennel and by one particular sire from that kennel in a four- generation pedigree predisposed for aggressiveness [24].

Gender
In an analysis of the caseload at the Ontario Veterinary College, although males were overrepresented among dogs that had dominance-related aggression as compared with dogs that had other behavior problems, neuter status had no influence. Guy and colleagues [26] showed that intact females were least likely to have bitten, and neutered males were most likely to have bitten. Among small breeds, being a female was a significant risk factor for biting, although this finding may have been a sampling effect rather than a true gender effect. Aggressive behavior of males occurred in more contexts and was considered more frightening by owners. This finding might be an additional reason males are more likely to be referred to a behavior specialist [29].

Reisner and colleagues [24] identified being male and being neutered (in either sex) as risk factors for biting.

Age
Of the cases analyzed at the Ontario Veterinary College, more than 50% of dogs started to exhibit "dominance-related aggression" at less than 1 year of age, and many exhibited this behavior as young as 3 to 4 months of age. Guy and colleagues [26] found that many dogs with aggression toward household members had growled over their food by the age of 2 months. At Purdue University, more than 70% of dogs had started to be aggressive by 1 year of age, and about 40% had begun to be aggressive by the age of 6 months. These findings are inconsistent with the traditional view of dominance-related aggression. Reisner and colleagues [24], however, found that being more than 4 years old was a risk factor in English Springer Spaniels.

Body language
Clients often report that their dogs show ambivalent body language during an attack, that they tremble after an attack, and that they slink away and seem "remorseful" (ie, show appeasement behavior) shortly after an attack. During behavior consultations, dogs presenting for aggression toward owners often show signs of fear. Again, this finding is inconsistent with the dog's being dominant.

Owner interaction

Dogs that were obtained for breeding or showing had less owner-directed aggression, and dogs obtained mainly for exercise had less owner-directed aggression and were less likely to compete aggressively for attention. Dogs of first-time owners were more likely to show aggression toward their owners and were more fearful. First-time owners rated their dogs as more excitable and less obedient than did experienced owners [30].

Another study looked at a connection between owner personality and behavior problems [31]. The most relevant finding was that dogs of owners who had great anthropomorphic involvement with their dogs were more likely to show aggression toward family members and visitors, especially when patted or disturbed, and to demand attention. It might be that anthropomorphic relationships have little structure and, therefore, are inconsistent and unpredictable, possibly in turn leading to stress, anxiety, conflict, and aggression.

Disposition and other behavior

Dogs that show aggression toward their owners were more excitable and more fearful in the first 2 months they spent with the owner [29]. They are more likely to have had a serious illness in the first 4 months of life [32]. Dogs that are aggressive towards their owners get less exercise, are slow in reacting to commands, are more likely to pull on the lead, are more fearful of people, are more excitable, and are more likely to react to loud or high-pitched noises [25,33]. These dogs may show pronounced appeasement behavior toward their owners in various situations. Dominant behavior toward unfamiliar dogs and aggression toward household members do not seem to be correlated. Aggression toward household members often is associated with territorial aggression toward unfamiliar people.

Conclusion

To reiterate, most cases of aggression toward household members do not fit the traditional concept of "dominance-related aggression." By far the majority of cases start at a relatively young age. The affected dogs often have a history of early disease and of excitability and fearfulness as puppies. They also are more excitable and more fearful as adults. Their body language before an attack is ambivalent and indicates high arousal. After a bite, affected dogs often are anxious and act submissive. They are likely to show appeasement behavior to people in other situations and often are submissive to other dogs. Furthermore, aggressive dogs have lower brain serotonin, whereas dominant animals should have high brain serotonin and show little aggression.

Alternative explanation

The following alternative explanation for these cases is offered. Aggression may be manifested in puppyhood as play aggression, fear aggression, or as a conflict behavior (aggression is exhibited by many species in experimental situations that induce motivational conflict or frustration). Fear aggression and conflict- or frustration-induced aggressions are rewarded by the person's retreating and leaving the dog alone. (Play-related aggression is negatively punished by a person retreating, because the puppy wants to interact, and being ignored is a negative punishment. Play-related aggression therefore is less likely to be at the root of a persistent problem of aggression toward owners.) The puppy then learns that it can get itself out of any uncomfortable situation by being aggressive.

The aggression is reinforced by avoidance conditioning because the anticipated bad event does not occur or because uncertainty is ended. This type of aggression therefore also has been called "avoidance-motivated aggression" [34]. Behaviors reinforced in this manner are very persistent (ie, very resistant to extinction). Conditioning with negative reinforcement has an additional effect: as the animal learns that the strategy is successful, it loses its fear. Therefore, although initially aggression usually is defensive or ambivalent in nature, the aggression very quickly can turn to offensive aggression.

Some dogs are genetically quite aggressive (ie, they resort to aggression very quickly); others are not aggressive at all (aggression trait). Some dogs are very fearful; others are not fearful at all (shyness/boldness trait) [20]. Therefore, some dogs may resort to aggression when only slightly uncertain, whereas others would use aggression only when severely frightened.

For any animal, including humans, it is very stressful not to be able to predict what is going to happen or not to be able to control what is happening at the moment (ie, not having control over pleasant or aversive stimuli). To improve its well being, every animal strives to assume a certain degree of control and to maximize predictability [35]. Aggressive dogs may resort to aggression as a coping strategy [34]. Even though these dogs may not be truly fearful, they nonetheless are uncertain and therefore are anxious. They resort to aggression as their strategy to operate on the environment and achieve a predictable outcome—the frightening person backing off. These dogs present similarly to "dominant dogs" in the traditional sense, although their aggression probably has nothing to do with social order. Punishment is not likely to have a beneficial effect on the aggression in such cases and may make it worse [34]. It is conceivable that punishment, if it is severe enough, could suppress the aggression, but it does not address the cause of the aggression (ie, the dog's uncertainty in an inconsistent environment). The authors suspect that highly trainable dogs that also are genetically predisposed to aggression may be at particular risk for that type of aggression, because they have been selected for being motivated to exert control over their environment (a dog that does not care about controlling rewards is not easily trained).

This concept has profound implications. It calls for an interpretation of the social relationship between dogs and owners using a more sophisticated paradigm than the dominance–submissiveness relationship. It points out the inappropriateness of domination techniques so often applied to puppies and adult dogs. It implies that any form of punishment for these cases of aggression is counterproductive, even though in some cases punishment can suppress the aggressive behavior. It draws into question traditional approaches to diagnosis, especially ones focusing only on the aggression and the behavior at the time of presentation and ones relying on fixed diagnostic criteria. It points out the importance of considering the development of a behavioral problem and the disposition of an animal when making a diagnosis and of the choice of an appropriate treatment regimen. It leads away from the idea of "counterdomination" and instead compels the development of a new approach to the treatment of aggression directed toward familiar people.

TREATMENT OF CONFLICT-RELATED AGGRESSION

Treatment should address the way in which the dog is managed, the dog's basic disposition (eg, fearfulness), and the cause of conflict (eg, inconsistency) in the owner–dog interaction and the dog's environment.

A caseload analysis done at the Ontario Veterinary College showed that when dogs that were fed ad lib were switched to meal feeding the behavioral prognosis was improved. Twice per day feeding is therefore recommended. Exercise off the property reduces anxiety levels, and dogs that are exercised regularly were shown to have less of a problem with aggression [33]. Therefore, at least two daily walks off the property are recommended. Dogs with little training also are more likely to be aggressive [33], and training to some cues is important for control of the dog and for diffusing potentially dangerous situations. Training also encourages the practice of specific prescribed behavior modification exercises. The authors therefore always recommend training. Clicker training is especially helpful when dealing with these dogs; because it does not require proximity to or physical contact with the aggressive dog, confrontations between owner and dog can more easily be avoided. (For a review of clicker training, see [36].)

Next, the dog's basic disposition should be evaluated and addressed. Aggressive dogs frequently are fearful or hyperexcitable. In the treatment of conflict-related aggression, both fear and hyperexcitability are addressed, at least in part, through "ignoring" (many cases of hyperexcitability are conditioned at least in part through owner attention, but some dogs may not tolerate a change in the amount of attention given them by owners), through consistent owner-initiated interaction (training gives the animal control over its environment and increases self-confidence), and through behavior modification techniques such as systematic desensitization, counterconditioning, and response substitution. These last three behavior modification techniques may have to be used in situations in which the dog is only fearful as well as in situations in which the dog is aggressive.

Situations in which confrontations are likely should be avoided, because any confrontation may undermine treatment success made to this point. The dog may need to be crate trained and crated or trained to an exercise pen and confined except during behavior modification excises. (Proper training to the crate or exercise pen is important so that the owner can get the dog back into the crate or pen, without confrontation, fear, or anxiety.) Confinement also is indicated when the owners are afraid of the dog, when smaller children are involved, or when the owner is unable to avoid casual interactions with the dog. Toys or other assets that could trigger confrontations should be removed. It may be important to keep the dog from climbing on furniture, particularly if aggression occurred in a furniture-related context, either by verbal cue or by restriction from the furnished room (eg, with a baby gate). The dog should be re-introduced to such situations only in the context of systematic desensitization, counterconditioning, and response substitution.

The main reason for conflict resulting from owner-to-dog interaction is that the dog cannot predict what is going to happen, does not know what to expect, and does not have a response available that would be appropriate for the situation. Therefore, owners are instructed to avoid all casual interaction and to interact with the dog only in a cue-response-reward format. The owner initiates all interactions by giving a cue and then reinforcing the desired response. In some cases it may be useful to prompt the dog to perform the behavior (using a head halter and dragline or any other prompt that is safe), and then reinforce the behavior. Food obviously is pleasant and nonthreatening (unlike petting), relaxes the dog, and can be tossed from a distance if necessary.

This approach is not the same as nothing-in-life-is-free [37], which is intended by many trainers to make the dog dependent on the owner and "submissive" to the owner. Instead the training program described in the previous paragraphs is designed to assure that any interactions with the dog are consistent (ie, the focus is on the owner's behavior, not the dog's). It also teaches the dog to operate on the environment in a successful and appropriate way. Highly structured obedience exercises, especially ones that desensitize the dog to owner behavior perceived as threatening, are very useful [38]. They provide an opportunity for predictable owner–dog interactions, desensitization to owner behavior, and substitution of aggression with learned, appropriate responses such as sitting or going to a mat elsewhere in the room.

In many cases it is helpful to use a head halter with a leash attached. The head halter is placed on the dog (the dog first is taught to accept the halter through systematic desensitization and counterconditioning; see http://abrionline.org) so that the owner can control all aggression-inducing situations in a nonconfrontational, consistent way. No punishment, no choke chains, and no scolding are used. The dog's behavior is controlled by the owner, but in a humane way that does not increase anxiety or arousal. A head halter also assists the owner in training and walking the dog. (In some cases, as is true for any close interaction, placing a head halter may increase the risk of biting; in these cases a head halter should not be used.)

When it is safe to do so, situations in which the dog still shows aggression are addressed by systematic desensitization and response substitution. The principle of systematic desensitization is to expose the dog gradually to a threatening or conflict-associated situation (eg, the owner "standing over" the dog) and to reward the dog for relaxation. Response substitution can be used to teach a dog to perform appropriate instead of inappropriate behavior. The head halter is an effective tool for preventing inappropriate behavior and to induce desired behavior that then can be rewarded. For example, when the dog is on the couch and growls when approached, the owner can pick up the indoor leash attached to the head halter, tell the dog to come, gently but firmly pull the dog off the couch, walk the dog away from the couch, ask it to sit, and reward. Again, the halter and leash are there to induce desired behavior so it can be rewarded, not to discipline or dominate the dog. The dog thus learns an alternative, acceptable, and stress-free way out of a conflict-inducing situation. Again, when such interactions increase the risk of biting, it may be necessary to avoid such situations altogether. For example, dogs that cannot be asked safely to get off furniture should be gated securely from the furnished room at all times.

It may not be possible or safe to desensitize a dog to all human–dog interactions. For example, there may not be a need for the dog to learn to accept "standing over" by the owner, and such exercises would be contraindicated.

Aggression Over the Food Bowl

A common situation in which dogs may show aggression is over their food. Although food-guarding behavior probably is a variant of normal behavior in dogs, it is unwanted and potentially dangerous. Food bowl aggression can be addressed by simple management. The food bowl is put down in a room with the door closed, while the dog is outside the room. The owner then leaves the room and sends the dog in to eat with the door securely closed. Once the dog is finished eating, the owner calls the dog back out of the room, goes in, closes the door, and picks up the food bowl and removes it. If children are in the home, the location in which the dog eats should be securely closed, perhaps with a latch placed high on the door or in a crate, to avoid the possibility of disturbing the dog inadvertently. In some cases it also is desirable to confine the dog while food is being prepared.

In some situations when owners willing to work with the dog, food-associated aggression can be addressed with a desensitization procedure as an optional intervention. Again, such exercises may introduce unnecessary risk; cases should be evaluated individually, and owners should be counseled carefully about safety. Owners are instructed to feed the dog in a different place and to use a different food bowl, preferably an old saucepan with a long handle, so that the dog does not associate feeding with previous confrontations. The dog should be tied for safety. The usual amount of food is to be measured out. Only three kibbles are to be placed into the food bowl (saucepan) at once. The dog is then asked to sit, and the food bowl is lowered so the dog can eat the kibbles while the owner continues to hold the saucepan by the handle. When the dog is finished eating, it is asked to sit again, the container is raised, and the procedure is repeated until all the food is consumed. If the dog shows any aggression at any time, the owner removes the saucepan and leaves the dog for 10 minutes. The procedure then is repeated. Once both owner and dog are comfortable with this procedure, the owner can start gradually to place more food into the saucepan. The next step is to go back to only three kibbles but to let go of the bowl's handle for short, and then increasingly longer, times. Once this process goes well, the owner again can increase the amount of food gradually. Eventually, the owner can place a third of the ration into the bowl and add more food with a ladle while the dog is eating. Finally, all the food can be placed into the bowl at once, and the owner can add strong-smelling treats such as small pieces of cheese or hot dogs to the feed while the dog is eating. In this way most dogs accept the owner's presence while eating. Progress must be monitored carefully, and with some dogs it may be unsafe to proceed to the last stages of this procedure. The authors do not recommend trying to touch the dog while it is eating, although with some dogs it may be possible to apply a desensitization procedure to achieve this behavior as well.

Guarding Items

Another situation in which conflict-related aggression often is exhibited is over stolen items or toys. In this situation the aggression often is called "resource guarding" or "possessive aggression," but in many cases it is conflict-related aggression in a specific context.

Dogs naturally guard resources. Seeing a pet devour a piece of chicken it dug out of the trash before someone can take it away or coveting a valued chew toy is a common sight to dog owners. Dogs also may guard objects such as socks, facial tissues, or plastic wrappers. In fact in many cases, the aggression seems to be related less to the item than to an expected confrontation, or to the owner's leaning down over or reaching toward the dog.

Resource guarding or possessive aggression can be very severe and quite dangerous to the owner. Such aggression expresses itself as guarding of an item from people or other animals. Possessive aggression commonly is related to conflict-induced aggression: possessive aggression in a puppy is a risk factor for aggression toward household members later in life [25]. Possessive aggression often is enhanced through inadvertent reinforcement by the owner: for example, some puppies become afraid when the owner wants to take an item away and run or hide under a bed (ie, they are cornered). When the owner reaches for them, they show fear-related aggression. The owner backs off, and the aggressive behavior is reinforced negatively. Other puppies get an item and enjoy the resulting "game" when the owner tries to catch them. Their behavior is reinforced positively by the owner's reaction.

It helps to teach a dog that giving up a stolen or valued object is not so bad because in return the dog will receive an extra special treat or maybe even a new toy. If a dog has learned that having things taken away is a very good thing, relinquishing items will not be a big deal; actually, the dog even may begin to look forward to it.

The basic exchange exercise

Precautionary safety instructions. To prevent further conflict while teaching the release command, it is best to keep all valuable items out of the dog's reach. If not all objects can be removed, and the dog still has the opportunity to grab objects and defend them, a head halter can be placed on the dog with a dragline attached. If the dog gets hold of an object, the owner can toss a very desirable treat some distance from the dog. The dog probably will drop the object and go over to the treat. The owner lets the dog take the treat but then leads the dog away from the stolen object. The stolen object is retrieved only after the dog is securely confined elsewhere. This technique should be attempted only by adults, not by children.

Exercises to practice basic exchange. With the dog in a down-stay and tied to an immovable object by its regular collar and away from the place in which it historically has shown aggression, the handler starts by showing the dog an object that the dog does not value much. The object is placed about 3 feet away from the dog; a release cue (eg, "off," or "leave-it") is given, and object is removed. The dog then is given a food reward, and the object is placed about 2.5 feet in front of the dog. Again, after the release cue is given, the object is removed, and the dog is rewarded for staying in a relaxed down-stay. As long as the dog is quiet and does not lunge for the object, the object is placed closer and closer to the dog, the release cue is given, the object is removed, and the dog is rewarded. The exercise is repeated with objects of increasing value to the dog. When highly desirable objects are used, the value of the treats must be increased as well.

Once the dog behaves well in these situations, the owner should leave out items that the dog will take in its mouth but that are not of high value to the dog. In such situations, the owner can practice exchanges with objects the dog has taken spontaneously. The owner may have to show the dog a treat as a prompt to release the object, pick up the object while giving the dog a treat, and then return the object to the dog. If that goes well, the owner can start to leave out objects of increasing value to the dog and keep practicing exchanges with these.

After successful completion of this exercise, it is important to run occasional "cold trials." When the dog is chewing on its favorite chew toy, the owner should go over to the dog, give the release cue, reward the dog for releasing the object with a highly valued treat, then return the toy to the dog. This exercise may not be safe with some dogs.

To make the dog feel comfortable releasing its favorite chew toy or stolen objects to any one and in any situation, new people who will handle the dog must follow the same protocol with the dog (each time starting at the beginning). The exercise also should be done in various locations, starting away from the place to which the dog usually retreats with a stolen item (often under a piece of furniture) and gradually moving closer to that place. Again, the exercise needs to be started from the beginning in each new location.

Another very effective method for treatment of resource guarding is to teach a release cue using clicker training [36,39]. Initially, the dog learns that the "click," a meaningless sound, means a food treat is coming (ie, the click becomes a conditions stimulus). Then the owner observes the dog picking up toys or other objects at home. As soon as the dog drops the toy, the owner clicks and treats. Soon, the dog will start to enjoy that game and pick up toys, look at or come over to the owner, and drop the toy, expecting a treat. At this point the owner will be able to predict when the dog is going to drop the toy and thus can give a cue just before that happens. Then, the owner occasionally does not give the release cue and then also does not reward the dog for dropping the object. (The cue must be given very frequently in the beginning, or the behavior of dropping toys will extinguish.) In addition, the owner uses the cue occasionally when the dog does not seem about to drop the toy and rewards the dog for successfully dropping it. In this way the dog learns to drop an object on cue and that dropping an object "pays off" only if the cue was given.

As in the exchange exercises, the owner then should leave some items of little value to the dog lying around and gradually increase the value of these items. The consistent interaction that this exercise provides also is helpful in eliminating conflict caused by an ambiguous type of relationship between owner and dog (see the previous discussion under conflict-induced aggression).

Some trainers use separate commands for leaving an object that the dog has yet not picked up and for dropping an object. It seems that the dog simply learns not to be in contact with a particular item. If only one command is used (often the word "off"), it generalizes to many other situations, such as the dog standing up on a person, scratching on the door, sniffing an unfamiliar but nervous dog, and so on.

Pharmacologic Treatment of Conflict-Related Aggression

Pharmacologic therapy often can facilitate behavior modification greatly. (See the earlier discussion of neurophysiology and the pharmacology of aggression.) The most commonly used drug is fluoxetine [8], a selective serotonin re-uptake inhibitor. It increases serotonergic transmission at the synapses and the activity of serotonin as a neurohormone. As a consequence, it also down-regulates serotonin receptors. Because of the complex nature of its pharmacologic effects, fluoxetine may take more than 4 weeks for full clinical effect. Fluoxetine has anxiolytic effects and is thought to also have antiaggressive properties. Sometimes fluoxetine can be combined with other drugs, either to reduce its most common side effect (reduced appetite) or to add a mood-stabilizing effect. Presently no medications are approved for the treatment of aggression in dogs.

Tryptophan supplementation of a low-protein diet also has been suggested as part of the treatment for owner-directed aggression [10], but the effect is inconsistent and therefore it seldom is used. In addition, the dog-appeasement pheromone (DAP, Ceva Santé Animale, Libourne Cedex, France) could be used as an adjunct treatment to reduce anxiety.

Punishment and Flooding

The considerations discussed previously lead to the conclusion that the use of punishment or flooding (uncontrolled exposure to the frightening stimulus) is contraindicated. Why do these techniques sometimes work? Some cases, there probably is not much fear or anxiety involved. Highly trainable dogs that are strongly motivated to operate on the environment to achieve predictable outcomes and at the same time are genetically highly predisposed for aggression may resort to aggression very quickly. The aggression is reinforced with negative reinforcement and by the dog's success in controlling the environment. In these cases, the main cause for the aggression may be conditioning (learned behavior), and behaviors that are largely learned are more amenable to change. If such a dog is punished for aggression, the aggression is suppressed; if, at the same time, the dog is taught appropriate behavior in the situation, it is taught an alternative coping strategy. Again, this approach is acceptable (but unnecessary and perhaps inhumane) if little anxiety is involved. Such cases are difficult or impossible to identify, however. Furthermore, the ability to apply the technique properly is low, and therefore the risks associated with applying this technique are unacceptably high. The currently proposed treatment strategies achieve similar results, albeit more gradually, without the high risk and detrimental effects on the dog's welfare.

PROGNOSIS

The prognosis for cases of canine aggression is worse than for most other behavior problems. Behaviorists generally give a guarded prognosis because there always is a risk that a dog might be aggressive again. The prognosis depends on the size of the dog, whether children are involved [40], whether the dog shows a graduated aggressive response (gives warning and escalates slowly) or an all-or-nothing response, and whether the dog has shown bite inhibition.

PREVENTION

Aggression in adult dogs may result from experiences and the environment early in life Examples include

- Lack of environmental stimulation
- Lack of handling
- Early weaning (possibly)
- Health issues
- Lack of socialization, exposure, and desensitization
- Inconsistent rules, environment, and interactions
- Adverse experiences, especially during the fear periods
- Lack of learning a bite inhibition, often because of lack of opportunity
- Lack of training

Addressing all these points allows a puppy raiser to diminish the chance that a genetically sound puppy might develop into an aggressive adult dog. Of course, training to prevent other behavior problems is just as important. For instance, a relaxed down-stay is useful in many situations, especially where the dog is either excitable or anxious; "alone training" is important in the prevention of separation anxiety; and housetraining of course is essential to allow a dog to share living quarters with its human family.

> **Box 1: Treatment of conflict-related aggression**
>
> 1. Management
>   Avoid confrontations (confinement, use head halter and leash, ignore dog)
>   Restrict feeding to twice a day (remove bowl after feeding)
>   Exercise off the property twice a day
>   Obedience training to command control
> 2. Temperament
>   Address fearfulness
>   Address hyperexcitability
> 3. Behavior modification
>   Avoid casual interactions
>   All interactions to be in a command-response-reward format
>   Counterconditioning (classical conditioning)
>   Response substitution
>   Systematic desensitization
> 4. Pharmacologic intervention (optional)
>   Fluoxetine, 1 to 2 mg/kg once a day

SUMMARY OF TREATMENT OF CONFLICT-RELATED AGGRESSION

Box 1 summarizes the treatment of conflict-related aggression.

When drugs are used as part of a treatment program for behavior problems, the authors suggest that practitioners read the article in this issue by Seibert and any listed references. For drugs that are not licensed for veterinary use, doses, indications, side effects, and contraindications may not have been studied adequately. Practitioners should be familiar with the published literature and dispense these medications with informed consent.

APPENDIX 1
CLIENT INFORMATION ON CONFLICT-RELATED AGGRESSION
Cause of Conflict-Related Aggression

Conflict-related aggression traditionally has been referred to as "dominance aggression" by most behaviorists. Dominance aggression is defined as aggression directed toward household members in situations in which the social position of the dominant dog is threatened. Most dogs seen for "dominance aggression" are not dominant or confident dogs, however. Instead, these dogs often act uncertain, fearful, or submissive. Owners often report that the dog shows ambivalent body language during and after an attack. These dogs may "slink off" after an attack, shake or show appeasement behaviors, or appear "remorseful" to the owner. Most dogs that are aggressive toward household members are not dominant, nor do they have confident personalities.

Affected dogs may become aggressive when they are in a conflict situation. Many conflicts occur when a dog cannot predict what is going to happen because of inconsistencies in dog–owner interactions. The dog is placed into a motivational conflict in these situations. It may want to be near the owner but also may be uneasy about what is going to happen. Another reason for a dog's showing aggression as a conflict behavior is that the environment is inconsistent and thus unpredictable, so that the dog feels it has no control over events. Unpredictability and lack of control over events are major stress factors for dogs, as well as for people. Although some dogs may be perfectly happy letting things happen around them as they may, others may become anxious if they cannot keep things under control. It has been hypothesized that this trait can be selected for inadvertently when selecting for trainability. Some have suggested that a dog that is highly trainable strongly desires control and predictability in its environment and interactions. Depending on their genetic make-up, these dogs may be quick to resort to aggression.

Affected dogs learn to use aggression as a coping mechanism and to exert some control over the environment (because the outcome of the aggression is predictable). The aggression is reinforced because the anticipated event that the dog fears does not occur or because the dog gains some control over the situation. For example, the owner approaches, and the dog is unsure of what is expected of it; it shows aggression to control the situation, and the owner backs off. The dog's aggressive behavior has been rewarded, because the dreaded event did not occur and it achieved a predictable outcome. Unfortunately, behaviors reinforced in this manner are very persistent.

Treatment of Conflict-Related Aggression

Because there are many different types of aggression that can be directed toward the owner, a behaviorist needs to make a specific diagnosis and devise a treatment plan appropriate for the individual case. The following techniques often are used in the treatment of conflict-related aggression.

Treatment should address the dog's basic disposition (eg, fearfulness, anxiety), the way in which the dog is managed, and the cause of conflict (eg, inconsistency) in the owner–dog interactions.

1. Avoid confrontation. The situations in which confrontations are likely should be avoided. Any confrontation may destroy the progress made to that point in treatment. The dog needs to be crate trained and crated or confined in an exercise pen unless being worked with. Confinement is indicated if the owners are afraid of the dog, if small children are involved, or if the owner is unable to ignore the dog. Toys and other assets that can cause confrontations should be removed. The dog is not to be allowed on the furniture, including the bed, if it has shown aggression in these situations in the past.

2. Use a head collar. The dog should wear a head collar with a dragline attached when the owners are home. A head collar allows the owner to diffuse any aggression-inducing situations in a nonconfrontational and consistent manner. Example: The dog has been aggressive when approached while on its bed. The owner may call the dog, use the head collar and dragline

to encourage the dog to "come," ask the dog to "sit," and then reward the dog. The confrontation (conflict) is avoided, and an appropriate and acceptable response is rewarded. If a head collar cannot be placed on the dog, a body harness may be an acceptable, although less effective, alternative.

3. The head collar or body harness also may be useful for walking and training the dog. Regular exercise (twice daily) helps reduce the dog's reactivity and anxiety.

4. Avoid inconsistent owner–dog interactions. The main reason for conflict resulting from owner-to-dog interaction is that the dog cannot predict what is going to happen and does not know what to do to achieve a predictable outcome. Therefore, owners are instructed to avoid all casual interactions with the dog and to interact in a command-response-reward format only. This procedure assures that any interactions with the dog are consistent and predictable. The owner gives a command; the dog responds and is rewarded for performing the behavior.

5. Structured obedience exercises. Nonconfrontational obedience training such as clicker training and the use of a head collar provides an opportunity for predictable owner–dog interaction, desensitizes the dog to owner behavior, and allows the owner to substitute appropriate responses for aggression. Obedience training using positive reinforcement also will have a long-lasting effect on the owner's behavior toward the dog by making it more consistent and confident. Obedience training allows the owner to tell the dog what to do before the dog makes the wrong choice (aggression), and the dog learns how to respond to achieve a predictable and desirable outcome.

6. Clicker training. Clicker training is especially appropriate for teaching aggressive dogs because it can be performed without contact and therefore is extremely nonconfrontational. With clicker training, appropriate behaviors can be "captured" and subsequently be put on cue. Training should be done in a no-nonsense attitude, upbeat but not playfully.

7. Do not use punishment. Punishment is contraindicated in treating aggression. No punishment of any type should be applied. Choke collars, pinch collars, verbal reprimands, or physical punishment are contraindicated in treating aggression. Punishment almost always is administered inconsistently and increases anxiety and fear. Punishment and domination techniques occasionally can be successful and yield very quick results, but their use is much too risky, both for the dog and for the owner. Furthermore, they tend to result not in the dog's being relaxed and happy but in its being in a state of learned helplessness.

8. Observe consistent and absolute rules. If the rules change all the time, the dog never can figure them out and cannot use them to control the environment. There should be a consistent rule structure that allows the dog to achieve a predictable outcome of its behavior and in which the behavior desired by the owner also pays off for the dog.

9. Apply behavior modification for specific situations: Specific situations in which the dog shows aggression may be addressed by gradually exposing the dog to the threatening or conflict situation (eg, the owner "standing over" the dog or touching specific areas on the dog) and rewarding the dog for relaxation. A previously threatening situation can be associated with a pleasant event (eg, giving the dog attention and petting only when

the owner touches a previously sensitive body part). An appropriate behavior can be substituted for a previously inappropriate behavior (eg, teaching the dog to "shake hands" to have its feet handled, with reward for the appropriate behavior).

References

[1] Landsberg G, Hunthausen W, Ackerman L. Handbook of behavior problems of the dog and cat. 2nd edition. Saunders (NY): Oxford; 2003. p. 385.

[2] Coppinger R, Coppinger L. Differences in the behavior of dog breeds. In: Grandin T, editor. Genetics and the behavior of domestic animals. London: Academic Press; 1998. p. 176–202.

[3] Goodwin D, Bradshaw JWS, Wickens SM. Paedomorphosis affects agonistic visual signals of domestic dogs. Anim Behav 1997;53:297–304.

[4] Boitani L, Francisci F, Ciucci P, et al. Population biology and ecology of feral dogs in central Italy. In: Serpell J, editor. The domestic dog, its evolution, behavior and interactions with people. Cambridge (UK): Cambridge University Press; 1995. p. 217–44.

[5] Bradshaw JWS, Nott HMR. Social and communication behaviour of companion dogs. In: Serpell J, editor. The domestic dog, its evolution, behavior and interactions with people. Cambridge (UK): Cambridge University Press; 1995. p. 115–30.

[6] Reisner IR, Mann JJ, Stanley M. Comparison of cerebrospinal fluid monoamine metabolite levels in dominant aggressive and non-aggressive dogs. Brain Res 1996;714:1–2.

[7] Bear MF, Connors BW, Paradiso MA. Neuroscience, exploring the brain. 3rd edition. Baltimore (MD): Lippincott Williams and Wilkins; 2007. p. 857.

[8] Dodman NH, Donnelly R, Shuster L, et al. Use of fluoxetine to treat dominance aggression in dogs. J Am Vet Med Assoc 1996;209:1585–7.

[9] White MM, Neilson JC, Hart BL, et al. Effects of clomipramine hydrochloride on dominance-related aggression in dogs. J Am Vet Med Assoc 1999;215.1288–91.

[10] DeNapoli JS, Dodman NH, Shuster L, et al. Effect of dietary protein content and tryptophan supplementation on dominance aggression, territorial aggression, and hyperactivity in dogs. J Am Vet Med Assoc 2000;217:504–8.

[11] Scott JP, Fuller JL. Dog behavior, the genetic basis. Chicago: The University of Chicago Press; 1965. p. 468.

[12] Cattell RB, Bolz CR, Korth B. Behavioral types in purebred dogs objectively determined by taxonome. Behav Genet 1972;3:205–16.

[13] Niimi Y, Inoue-Murayama M, Murayama Y, et al. Allelic variation of the D4 dopamine receptor polymorphic region in two dog breeds, Golden Retriever and Shiba. J Vet Med Sci 1999;61(12):1281–6.

[14] Niimi Y, Inoue-Murayama M, Kato K, et al. Breed differences in allele frequency of the dopamine receptor D4 gene in dogs. J Hered 2001;92(5):433–6.

[15] Ito H, Nara H, Inoue-Murayama M, et al. Allele frequency distribution of the canine dopamine receptor D4 gene exon III and I in 23 breeds. J Vet Med Sci 2004;66(7):815–20.

[16] Hart BL, Hart LA. Selecting pet dogs on the basis of cluster analysis of breed behavioral profiles and gender. J Am Vet Med Assoc 1985;186:1181–5.

[17] Bradshaw JWS, Goodwin D. Determination of behavioural traits of pure-bred dogs using factor analysis and cluster analysis; a comparison of studies in the USA and UK. Res Vet Sci 1998;66:73–6.

[18] Svartberg K. Shyness-boldness predicts performance in working dogs. Appl Anim Behav Sci 2002;79(2):157–74.

[19] Svartberg K. A comparison of behaviour in test and in everyday life: evidence of three consistent boldness-related personality traits in dogs. Appl Anim Behav Sci 2005;91:103–28.

[20] Svartberg K, Forkman B. Personality traits in the domestic dog (canis familiaris). Appl Anim Behav Sci 2002;79:133–55.

[21] Strandberg E, Jacobsson J, Saetre P. Direct genetic, maternal and litter affects on behaviour in German shepherd dogs in Sweden. Livestock Production Science 2004;93:33–42.

[22] Van den Berg L. Genetics of aggressive behavior in golden retriever dogs [thesis]. Utrecht (NL): Utrecht University; 2006. p. 215–20.

[23] Podberscek AL, Serpell JA. The English Cocker Spaniel: preliminary findings on aggressive behaviour. Appl Anim Behav Sci 1996;47:75–89.

[24] Reisner IR, Houpt KA, Shofer FS. National survey of owner-directed aggression in English Springer Spaniels. J Am Vet Med Assoc 2005;227:1594–603.

[25] Guy NC. Canine household aggression in the caseload of general veterinary practitioners in Maritime Canada [MSc thesis]. Charlottetown (PE): University of PEI; 1999. p. 186.

[26] Guy NC, Luescher UA, Dohoo SE, et al. Demographic and aggressive characteristics of dogs in a general veterinary caseload. Appl Anim Behav Sci 2001;74:15–28.

[27] O'Farrell E, Peachey E. Behavioural effects of ovariohysterectomy on bitches. J Small Anim Pract 1990;31:595–8.

[28] Heath S. Medical differential diagnosis—what needs to be considered. Presented at the meeting of the Norwegian Veterinary Association. Oslo (Norway), March 30–April 1, 2000.

[29] Guy NC, Luescher UA, Dohoo SE, et al. Risk factors of dog bites to owners in a general veterinary caseload. Appl Anim Behav Sci 2001;74:29–42.

[30] Jagoe A, Serpell J. Owner characteristics and interactions and the prevalence of canine behaviour problems. Appl Anim Behav Sci 1996;47:31–42.

[31] O'Farrell V. Owner attitudes and dog behaviour problems. Appl Anim Behav Sci 1997;52:205–13.

[32] Serpell J, Jagoe JA. Early experience and the development of behavior. In: Serpell J, editor. The domestic dog, its evolution, behavior and interactions with people. Cambridge (UK): Cambridge University Press; 1995. p. 79–102.

[33] Podberscek AL, Serpell JA. Environmental influences on the expression of aggressive behavior in English Cocker Spaniels. Appl Anim Behav Sci 1997;52:215–27.

[34] Tortora DF. Safety training: the elimination of avoidance-motivated aggression in dogs. Aust Vet Pract 1984;14:70–4.

[35] Wiepkema PR. Abnormal behaviors in farm animals: ethological implications. Netherlands Journal of Zoology 1985;35:279–99.

[36] Pryor K. Clicker training for dogs. Waltham (MA): Sunshine Books, Inc.; 1999. p. 52.

[37] Voith VL, Borchelt PL. Diagnosis and treatment of dominance aggression in the dog. Vet Clin North Am Small Anim Pract 1982;12(4):655–63.

[38] Overall KL. Clinical behavioral medicine for small animals. St. Louis (MO): Mosby; 1997. p. B–1 and B–3.

[39] Tillman P. Clicking with your dog: step-by-step in pictures. Waltham (MA): Sunshine Books, Inc.; 2000. p. 209.

[40] Reisner IR, Erb HN, Houpt KA. Risk factors for behavior-related euthanasia among dominant-aggressive dogs: 110 cases (1989–1992). J Am Vet Med Assoc 1994;205:855–63.

Vet Clin Small Anim 38 (2008) 1131–1143

VETERINARY CLINICS
SMALL ANIMAL PRACTICE

Human-Directed Aggression in the Cat

Terry Marie Curtis, DVM

College of Veterinary Medicine, University of Florida, P.O. Box 100126, Gainesville, FL 32610, USA

S tudies indicate that aggression is second only to inappropriate elimination for feline cases seen by veterinary behavior specialists [1]. Although aggression is a normal component of the cat's behavioral repertoire [2], when directed toward the human caregiver it can result in injury and put a strain on the human–animal bond. The consequence could be resultant substandard care of the cat, relinquishment, or even euthanasia. Not all aggression is the same, so the motivation on the part of the cat needs to be taken into account when diagnosing and treating the problem. Motivation usually can be determined by the context as well as the cat's body posture and any vocalizations. A cat that is crouching and hissing with its ears back is exhibiting fear, whereas the cat that appears more erect with its ears up and forward is displaying confidence [2].

Any underlying medical condition that results in pain or discomfort can contribute to irritability and a subsequent aggression problem. Therefore, a thorough physical examination and any pertinent medical testing should be conducted as part of the comprehensive work-up of any feline aggression problem. Historical information is of utmost importance and includes the household environment, interactions between the cat and its human(s), feeding schedule, play and grooming routines, and other considerations. Whether the cat lives only indoors or has access to the outside should be determined. Outdoor stimuli have been implicated in cases of feline aggression [3], particularly redirected aggression [4]. Once the diagnosis is made, the treatment plan should be formulated to address the individual cat, the individual owner, and the household particulars. For example, the recommendations for a cat that has fear-motivated aggression and lives in a household with one adult caretaker are going to be quite different than those for the one living in a household with three other cats, two dogs, two adults, and three young children.

The more common categories of human-directed aggression include play, fear, petting intolerance, redirected aggression, pain, and maternal aggression. Status-related aggression and sexually motivated aggression also are sometimes seen, but not all veterinary behaviorists agree on these diagnostic categories.

E-mail address: curtist@mail.vetmed.ufl.edu

0195-5616/08/$ – see front matter
doi:10.1016/j.cvsm.2008.04.009

PLAY-MOTIVATED AGGRESSION

Play-motivated aggression is most common in younger cats but can be seen at any age. It usually, but not necessarily, is directed toward moving stimuli, and it may be directed only toward some members (both human and animal) of the household. Why certain individuals are chosen is not clear. In play, the cat approaches its victim, crouches in wait, stalks, and chases, with tail twitching and a focused stare. The ears are forward, not back, and generally the cat is silent. Play-motivated aggression directed toward people may be seen in orphan-reared cats that have no littermates or other cats to play with that both serve as an outlet for play and help the kitten learn how to inhibit play appropriately [5]. The results of a study conducted by Chon [6], however, showed that hand-reared cats are no more likely to display human-directed aggression and fear and are no more likely to develop behavior problems than queen-raised kittens and, in fact, are significantly friendlier to people. The presence of another cat in the household and the use of a wand-type toy were shown to decrease the likelihood of aggression toward people. Other possible predisposing factors for play-motivated aggression may be a history of using hands or feet to play with the kitten, playing roughly with the kitten, and/or inadequate opportunity for acceptable play. Although the motivation for the cat's aggression is playful, the cat often is referred to as "vicious." The victim may incur serious injury, including deep bite wounds and/or serious scratches. In short, this playfully motivated behavior can be very frightening and injurious to the victim.

Treatment

When possible, avoiding situations that elicit the behavior is a prudent strategy. If the owner is unsure when or where the problem behavior occurs, a journal may help identify times and places and facilitate avoidance strategies. The cat quickly learns what situations result in the play that it is seeking. In some cases the treatment can be as easy as having the "victim" enter through a different door or not wearing particular clothes (eg, flowing skirts, loose trousers) that cause the cat to engage in the behavior. The cat can be put in another room during times when the problem is likely to be worse (eg, when the owner is preparing dinner or working at a desk). It is important at that time to provide the cat with plenty of toys that are appropriate for the cat and acceptable to the owners, so that the separation is not viewed as punishment and the cat has the opportunity for appropriate play.

The owner must attempt to have daily opportunities for acceptable and appropriate play designed to meet the individual cat's needs. Depending on the type of toys the cat prefers, these sessions could involve dragging string, rolling balls, tossing small fuzzy mice, or other activities. The owner might tie a string to his or her body with an end that falls several feet away. A toy the cat enjoys is attached to the end of the string. This way, the cat and the owner can have interactive play, one hopes without injury to the owner.

The owner should be counseled to redirect the cat towards appropriate play whenever it seems to be in a playful mood and as early in the stalking sequence as possible. Keeping a daily diary might make it possible to schedule these play sessions so as to pre-empt the predatory play. It is useful to have a variety of toys available in multiple locations. Interactive toys that do not necessarily require the owner's presence can teach the cat how to play independently. There are cat trees that incorporate string toys into the design as well as a multitude of other options. Particular favorite interactive toys include any of the Cat Dancer (Arcata Pet Supplies, Arcata, California) and Panic Mouse (Panic Mouse, Inc, Torrance, California) products.

Appropriate interactive punishment can be implemented, because the situations usually allow the three components that are required for punishment to be effective [7]. First, the punishment must be immediate, occurring within a few seconds of the behavior. Second, the punishment must be consistent, happening every time that the behavior occurs. These two conditions can be met because the owner is always present when the play-motivated aggression occurs. The third condition is that the punishment must be appropriate, so that the behavior ceases but the cat does not become afraid of its owner. Examples include a "shhsst" sound, spraying a water pistol, or shaking a can of treats. The goal is to interrupt the sequence so that the cat then can be directed to more appropriate playful behavior. Physical punishments by the owner must be avoided because they can cause fear, anxiety, and even defensive aggression.

This is one case in which another cat—or even two—may be very helpful in resolving the problem, especially if the owner has expressed the desire for another cat. Adding another cat to the household may provide an outlet for normal and appropriate feline play. Adopting a juvenile cat rather than an adult would be recommended, because it would be more likely to play and would be easier, overall, to incorporate into the household [8]. Medications rarely are indicated in cases of play-motivated aggression because it is a normal behavior directed toward an inappropriate target. If the cat is particularly aroused and subsequently anxious, however, short-term treatment with a medication to help decrease anxiety and arousal may be beneficial (Table 1). Pharmacologic is discussed later in this article.

Table 1 Feline medications	
Medication	Oral dose for cats
Fluoxetine	0.5–1.5 mg/kg every 24 hours
Paroxetine	0.5–1.5 mg/kg every 24–48 hours
Sertraline	0.5–1.5 mg/kg every 24 hours
Clomipramine	0.25–1.3 mg/kg every 24 hours
Amitriptyline	0.5–2.0 mg/kg every 12–24 hours
Buspirone	2.5–7.5 mg/cat every 12–24 hours or 0.5–1.0 mg/kg every 12–24 hours

FEAR-RELATED AGGRESSION

Fear-related aggression also is a common cause of feline aggression directed at people. A fearful cat typically has its ears back and its body and tail lowered [2]. Generally the cat tends to avoid the person or persons at whom the aggression is directed, but in some cases the cat may attack the person. The aggression tends to occur when the cat is approached and/or reached for, especially when the cat is cornered and/or feels threatened. In some cases there may be a history of poor socialization or feral living, but fear-motivated aggression can occur in any cat, any breed, at any age, and in either sex, regardless of neuter status, and may have a genetic component as well. Often, fear-related aggression is the result of classical conditioning in which the cat associates the presence of a certain person with an aversive event. For example, a loud noise occurs in the presence of someone in the household. The cat runs and hides and subsequently may be reluctant to engage with that particular person. The target of the cat's aggression may remain directed at that one person, or the cat may begin to generalize and show fear in response to all men, all women, all children, or even all people except for a core few. In some cases the inciting stimulus can be identified; in other situations it is unknown or not remembered by the owner.

Treatment

The goal of treatment is to change the relationship and cat's perception of the person it fears. The cat needs to learn that bad things never happen when that person is around, and in fact great things happen! The process must go slowly. The technique of desensitization and counterconditioning is used to accomplish this change. In the desensitization is te process the cat is exposed to a stimulus (frightening person) that elicits a given response (run, hide, hiss, attack), but the exposure is at such a low level that the response is not elicited [9]. The person must be far enough away so that the cat is not afraid. Over time and with successive repetitions, the intensity of the stimulus is increased gradually (ie, the distance between the cat and the person decreases), and the exposure should occur without eliciting the fearful response. This process allows the cat to learn that nothing bad happens when the "scary person" is around. Counterconditioning is a procedure that reverses the cat's fearful response to a stimulus (the "scary person") by associating the stimulus with an unconditioned stimulus that promotes the opposite type of reaction. What is desired is a response that is behaviorally and physiologically incompatible with the previous fearful response, working from the premise that the cat cannot be afraid and relaxed at the same time. Examples include sitting for food rewards and engaging in play. Therefore, in the presence of the "scary person," while the cat is relaxed, it is offered a particularly yummy food or is played with or groomed. The goal is to change a previously fear-inducing situation to one in which the underlying emotional affect is relaxed and positive.

The desensitization and counterconditioning process is highly individualized and is based on the particular inducements that are particularly motivating to the fear-aggressive cat. For example, for the cat that likes to chase string and/or a toy attached to a string, the target person can drag the string, starting at whatever distance is necessary for the cat to pursue. The length can be shortened gradually over many days. For cats that are more motivated by food, the target person can sit or stand at a distance such that the cat is not afraid. Food rewards should be selected that have high value to the cat. The person can toss treats to the cat, or someone can lay a "treat trail" to the person. Some cats will like the play aspect of tossing the treats paired with the food motivation. In other situations the target person can be present when the cat is offered a bowl full of highly palatable food. The distance between the person and the food bowl depends on how fearful the cat is and initially must be far enough so that the cat will approach the bowl and eat. Gradually, the person can be closer and closer to the bowl, as long as the cat continues to remain and eat without vocalization such as growling or hissing. If the cat leaves the area without eating, the person probably is too close, and the distance should be increased at the next feeding.

If the cat is afraid only of certain people, another option is to have the person who can handle the cat play with it and/or give it treats while a person the cat fears sits quietly nearby. The distance must be determined carefully and be far enough that the cat is relaxed. Over time, the person the cat fears gradually comes closer and closer and perhaps even can offer the cat treats or initiate play.

Medication may be necessary to decrease the cat's overall level of anxiety so that it will be relaxed enough to learn that the "scary person" is not dangerous. Pharmacologic options include the serotonin partial agonist buspirone, the selective serotonin reuptake inhibitors (SSRIs) fluoxetine, paroxetine, and sertraline, and the tricyclic antidepressants (TCAs) amitriptyline and clomipramine. Whenever medication is used, the goal is to use as low a dose as necessary to decrease the cat's anxiety. Ideally, after approximately 3 months of desirable behavior, the cat is weaned from the medication slowly (see Table 1 and the pharmacologic discussion later in this article) [10].

PETTING INTOLERANCE

Petting intolerance and the associated aggressive response occur in some cats when the owner initiates petting and/or after a certain amount of petting or physical contact. In such cases, the cat turns around and "attack." These attacks can be minor inhibited bites or multiple injurious bites. The consequences can be severe, especially if the punctures are deep. The exact cause of petting intolerance in cats is controversial. Cats primarily groom each other on the head and neck [11,12], so being groomed or petted on other parts of the body may contribute to this reaction in certain individuals. The cat usually signals its "displeasure" by twitching its tail and skin. The ears usually are back, and the cat may emit a hiss and/or low growl and then perhaps turn and bite the person who is touching it. The amount of interaction the cat tolerates before an aggressive response varies from cat to cat but may be relatively predictable in some individuals.

Treatment

In many cases the cats offer warning before the aggressive response. Therefore, owners need to be instructed to watch for the cues that petting-intolerant cats tend to give before they strike. They may not realize that the cues are happening or significant until they are pointed out: ears laid back, tail twitching, body tense, skin rippling, and mydriasis. Because avoidance of aggression is the first line of treatment, all interactions should cease at the very first sign of agitation. It may be beneficial to instruct the owners to pet the cat only on its head and neck, avoiding the back and tail areas that often elicit the aggressive response.

Many petting-intolerant cats have a time limit/threshold for petting or grooming, and with observation most owners can learn what that time limit/threshold is. The cat owner must cease interaction before the cat shows any of the signs of agitation. For example, if the cat starts showing preaggression cues as early as 30 seconds after the start of petting, the owner never should pet the cat for more than 20 to 25 seconds. The owner can couple the petting with offering the cat a yummy treat (counterconditioning) and gradually build up to longer and longer periods of petting. In general, it is important for the owner to engage in other positive activities with the cat besides petting, such as feeding treats or playing with a particularly desirable toy, and to respect the individual cat's need and desire for physical contact.

Medication can be used to facilitate positive interactions between the cat and its owner but is controversial. Buspirone has been reported to have the side effect of "increased affection" directed toward the owner [13], which is the exact goal in this case. In most cases, however, finding the type of interaction the cat enjoys and avoiding emotionally arousing interactions works quite well, and medication is rarely needed.

REDIRECTED AGGRESSION

Redirected aggression occurs during interference in situations that have caused the cat to become aggressively aroused, such as a cat fight (between familiar household cats) or the mere presence of a stray cat outside. If the cat is denied access to the primary target, the aggressive behavior is redirected onto another, often closer, target. This form of feline aggression can result in severe injury (Fig. 1A, B) and can put a strain on cat–cat and cat–human relationships. In some cases, household cats may need to be re-introduced to each other because the relationship has been so damaged.

Treatment

It is important to address the primary problem (ie, the event or stimulus that caused the cat to become aggressively aroused in the first place), if that situation can be identified. If the cat in question is aroused by the presence of a stray cat outside, it may be as simple as denying the indoor cat access to the window either by using blinds or by closing the door. The use of a motion detector

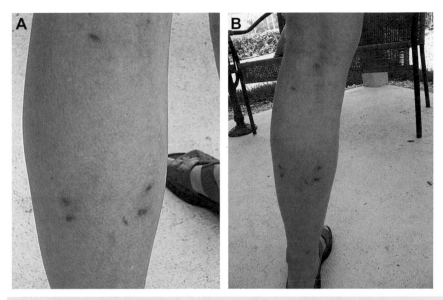

Fig. 1. (A and B) Leg of client showing feline bite marks from a redirected aggression event.

device such as the CatStop or Scarecrow (Contech Electronics, Inc., Victoria, British Columbia, Canada) may be effective in deterring the stray cat from coming onto the property in the first place.

In some situations the cat may become aroused aggressively by noises or odors, and these might be more difficult to avoid. If the problem occurs with visitors to the home or workmen, the cat should be confined before those situations take place.

For owner safety it is essential to avoid interacting with the cat if it already is aggressively emotionally aroused, because that is when the redirected behavior is most likely to occur. If possible, close the cat in a darkened room and allow it to calm down. Caution must be exercised when confining the cat, and the owner must be instructed to avoid picking up the cat but should "herd" the cat into the confinement location or cover the cat with a thick towel or blanket before picking it up.

Facilitate positive interactions between the affected cats in the household and/or between the cat and the owner by implementing more play time, providing rewards with favorite foods and treats, and incorporating more grooming sessions into the daily routine. These interactions must be initiated only after it is clear that the cat no longer is agitated and now is calm.

Medication may be necessary and is based on the level of the cat's arousal, the owner's attitude, and the primary cause of the aggression. If the cat is in a constant state of vigilance and agitation, medication could be very beneficial. If the owner is afraid of the cat and is considering re-homing or euthanasia, medication should be considered. If the primary cause—such as stray cats or other animals outside—cannot be managed completely, medication may be helpful. The SSRIs, partial serotonin agonists, or tricyclic antidepressants are recommended (see Table 1 and see pharmacologic discussion later in this article).

PAIN-RELATED AGGRESSION

Pain-related aggression can be associated with chronic conditions involving the eyes or ears, nail trims (too close to the quick), grooming (combing out mats), or any other medical conditions causing pain or discomfort: arthritis, bite wounds (subclinical abscesses), urinary tract infections, or a gastrointestinal foreign body, among others. With the more chronic painful conditions the cat may begin to generalize and become fearful of the person medicating it. Therefore, fear probably is one of the components of pain aggression, and the aggression must be treated accordingly.

Treatment

One should identify any medical conditions and treat them appropriately. For any on-going medical condition that requires regular treatment, one should attempt to make medicating the affected area a positive experience. If the cat is experiencing chronic pain, perhaps from arthritis, the underlying condition should be treated as well. For example, if the cat has recurring ear infections, one should warm the medication and avoid pouring it into the ear. Instead, the liquid should be applied to a cotton ball that is manipulated inside the ear by rubbing the ear gently. Using a series of wet-dry-wet-dry cotton balls, the ear can be kept clean and medicated in a more gentle way. If possible, one should not do all the medicating at one time unless it can be done very quickly and efficiently. One should employ the technique of classical conditioning and pair the medicating activity with a yummy treat. For example, giving the cat treats during its nail trim or grooming session can change the meaning of such an activity. In any case, it is important that the cat receive attention and interaction at times other than those involving a procedure and/or medication. Otherwise, the cat can learn that the owner is something to fear, and fear aggression may result.

MATERNAL AGGRESSION

Maternal aggression usually is predictable and self limiting. The queen, as part of her normal behavior, may protect her nest and kittens, especially from unfamiliar people. Avoidance is the strategy of choice, because a cornered queen can attack [14]. In the early stages of gestation, it is advisable to expose the queen to the people she is likely to encounter postpartum so that she is less likely to show aggression in the first place. Gradual desensitization and counterconditioning can be employed so that the queen associates good things with the presence of people. As the kittens mature, the aggressive behavior of the queen diminishes.

SEXUAL AGGRESSION

Sexual aggression is rare in cats. When it does occur, the cat showing the aggression usually is male, either intact or neutered [11]. This type of aggression manifests by the cat mounting the owner's limb, grabbing the skin, initiating pelvic thrusting, and growling. Although the queen has the protection of fur during the nape grip as part of the feline mating behavior, the human arm, in particular, is likely to be injured.

Treatment

It they are not being used for breeding, intact animals should be neutered. Punishment can be used and ideally should be implemented before the cat initiates the mounting sequence. A squirt bottle or other punisher should be used when the cat first focuses on the owner. Diffuse the behavior and redirect the cat toward more appropriate behavior, such as play. Some cats may be very anxious, and mounting behavior is a result of anxiety arising from other causes including poor environmental stimulation and poor control over consequences in the environment. If these issues are not addressed, mounting behavior may continue. See the article by Levine in this issue for information on feline fear and anxiety.

Medication can be used to decrease arousal, but no studies are available to assess its efficacy for this condition. The author has personal knowledge of one case responding very well to the TCA clomipramine, but the SSRIs also should be considered.

SOCIAL STATUS AGGRESSION

Status aggression is uncommon and controversial in cats, but many believe that it does occur. It usually is associated with attempts to make the cat do things it does not wish to do or to control a situation such as petting or moving the cat [15]. In such cases, the cat typically shows assertive displays to one or more persons in the household. Assertive posture is erect and stiff, with the ears up and rotated laterally. This posture is opposite of the crouched posture of the playful or fearful cat. It also is possible that this manifestation is a form of conflict-related aggression resulting from inconsistent and unpredictable owner responses. (See the article by Luescher and Reisner in this issue for a definition of conflict-related aggression in dogs).

Treatment

Status-related aggression can be managed by redirecting the cat toward more constructive activities, such as play. Medication may be necessary if the cat's level of arousal or reactivity is particularly high. It is also important to provide the opportunity for positive interactions and to reward the cat when it does interact with the owner in a nonaggressive manner. The cat also can be requested to perform a task before it obtains what it wants, can be given attention only when calm, and even can be taught tricks. The goal is for consequences to be predictable to reduce conflict and to help the cat learn more quickly which actions earn rewards and which do not.

Medication can be used to decrease the cat's reactivity but may not change the behavior appreciably without concurrent behavioral modification techniques. Pharmacologic options include the serotonin partial agonist buspirone, the SSRIs fluoxetine, paroxetine, and sertraline, and the TCAs amitriptyline and clomipramine (see Table 1 and the pharmacologic discussion later in this article).

PHARMACOLOGIC INTERVENTIONS
FOR HUMAN-DIRECTED AGGRESSION

Psychoactive medications can be useful in certain cases of human-directed aggression in cats, but it is rare for medication alone to provide a cure. In most cases, treatment is most effective if medication is used in combination with environmental management and behavioral modification, such as desensitization and counterconditioning. Psychoactive medications are used primarily to decrease the level of anxiety and reactivity in the cat so that learning can take place more effectively. For example, in fear-motivated aggression, it can take a long time for the cat to unlearn the negative association that it has with one or more persons. Use of an anxiolytic can facilitate a calmer demeanor and allow the cat to learn more quickly and effectively, allowing the desensitization and counterconditioning process to proceed faster. Medication use typically is short term. Doses are increased gradually to optimal levels, and ideally the cat is weaned from the medication when the time comes to do so. The drug classes commonly used for human-directed feline aggression are the SSRIs, the TCAs, the azapirones, and the benzodiazepines. A good general resource for the use of psychoactive medications in cats is *Veterinary Psychopharmacology* by Crowell-Davis and Murray [13]. None of the medications discussed in this section are approved for usage in cats, and informed owner consent is advisable before administration of any of these medications. In some cases blood work also may be prudent to assess the health of the animal treated.

The SSRIs are a class of antidepressants that have anxiolytic, anticompulsive, and some antiaggressive effects. Examples include fluoxetine (Prozac, Reconcile), paroxetine (Paxil), and sertraline (Zoloft). Inhibiting the reuptake of serotonin a results in an increase in serotonergic neurotransmission, allowing serotonin molecules to act for extended periods of time. The SSRIs typically are administered daily, not on an "as needed" basis. Although some response may be observed within a few days, improvement commonly does not occur for 3 to 4 weeks, or even longer. Therefore, it is important not to evaluate the pet's response to the medication until it has been given consistently for at least a month. Certainly, if any adverse effects are seen at any time, the dose should be decreased or use of the medication stopped entirely. Side effects observed in various species include sedation, tremor, constipation, diarrhea, nausea, anxiety, irritability, agitation, insomnia, decreased appetite, anorexia, aggression, mania, decreased libido, hyponatremia, and seizures. Mild sedation and decreased appetite are the most common side effects observed in cats. Some behaviorists have noted constipation and urine retention with paroxetine. In most cases the side effects seem to be dose dependent; therefore, starting at very low doses and working up to a maintenance dose that addresses the primary problem may diminish the occurrence of side effects.

The TCAs act as inhibitors of both serotonin and norepinephrine. They also have antihistaminic and anticholinergic effects and are α-adrenergic antagonists, which accounts for many of the side effects seen. Like the SSRIs, the TCAs have anxiolytic, anticompulsive, and antiaggressive effects. The TCAs vary in their ability to affect the increase of serotonin and as a class are not as serotonin-selective as the SSRIs. For example, amitriptyline (Elavil) has weak serotonin reuptake inhibition, but it is a strong antihistamine. Clomipramine (Anafranil, Clomicalm) is the most selective TCA for serotonin. The latency to effect is similar to that of the SSRIs, and therefore these medications also need to be given daily. To ameliorate gastric side effects (diarrhea, constipation, appetite changes), however, TCAs usually are administered twice daily as a divided dose. Other side effects include sedation, urinary retention, ataxia, decreased tear production, mydriasis, cardiac arrhythmias, tachycardia, and changes in blood pressure. To avoid overdosage and serotonin syndrome, TCAs and SSRIs should not be given together.

Azapirones are serotonin 1A agonists. They can be used for a variety of anxiety disorders and behaviors that may be affected by chronic anxiety, including general anxiety, urine marking, separation anxiety, and subordinate or timid cats that are the regular recipients of aggression. Buspirone (BuSpar) is the only azapirone that is commercially available in the United States. Side effects with buspirone are uncommon, which is one advantage to its use, although there are anecdotal reports of cats actually becoming more agitated on this medication rather than calmer. Several desirable side effects have been reported in cats, including owners' reports of their cats becoming "more affectionate." Cats that are not very social begin to exhibit some degree of social behavior. While the cat is on medication, it is capable of learning, and the social dynamic between cat and owner changes so that many cats retain increased levels of social behavior even after the medication is discontinued. Buspirone can be given in conjunction with TCAs and SSRIs; in combination, the doses of each are lowered accordingly.

Benzodiazepines work by facilitating gamma-aminobutyric acid in the central nervous system. They are anxiolytic medications with a rapid onset of action that lasts for a few to several hours, depending on the specific drug. Typically in cats the author has reserved the use of benzodiazepines—specifically, alprazolam—for cases of separation anxiety. Some cases of contextual (occurring only when the owner is out of town) overgrooming and urine marking have responded very well to this medication. Side effects typical of the benzodiazepines include sedation, ataxia, muscle relaxation, increased appetite, and paradoxical excitation. Benzodiazepines are Drug Enforcement Agency (DEA) Schedule IV drugs and have potential for human abuse. Reports of hepatotoxic reactions have been noted with diazepam, and this medication should be avoided when possible [16].

All the medications mentioned earlier are administered orally, which can be a problem for some cats. Having a daily handling ritual may add to the stress of any already anxious cat and owner, and that situation is not desirable. Some of the drugs, especially the TCAs, are very bitter, so it is important that the cat never taste them when they are administered. Pill Pockets (Fabrique par: S&M NuTec, LLC, North Kansas City, Missouri) have been use very successfully, especially in cats that like treats. Other ways to get a cat to take medication in food is to have the pill piece small enough and hidden in a pastelike vehicle such as cream cheese (salmon flavor is a particular favorite of many cats), whipped cream, ice cream, or cheese sauce or spread. The goal is for the cat to lick up the food and pill together and swallow it whole – without chewing. Although the idea of administering medication transdermally, especially to a fractious cat, is exciting, data available to date on psychotropic medications have shown the transdermal route of administration is ineffective. In a study by Mealey and colleagues [17], system absorption of amitriptyline and buspirone administered by the transdermal route was poor compared with that administered by the oral route. Likewise, in a study by Ciribassi and colleagues [18], the relative bioavailability of fluoxetine administered transdermally was only approximately 10% of that administered orally. That said, there have been anecdotal reports of transdermal administration of amitriptyline and fluoxetine being effective, but whether this is a drug effect or placebo effect is unknown. If all attempts at orally medicating the cat have failed, this avenue might be worth exploring.

When drugs are used as part of a treatment program for behavior problems, the Authors suggest that practitioners read the article in this issue by Seibert and any listed references. For drugs that are not licensed for veterinary use, doses, indications, side effects and contraindications may not be studied adequately; practitioners should be familiar with the published literature and dispense these medications with informed consent.

References

[1] Bamberger M, Houpt KA. Signalment factors, comorbitity and trends in behavioral diagnoses in cats: 736 cases 1991–2001. Journal of the American Veterinary Medical Association 2006;229(1):1602–6.

[2] Bradshaw J, Cameron-Beaumont C. The signalling repertoire of the domestic cat and its undomesticated relatives. In: Turner DC, Bateson P, editors. The domestic cat—the biology of its behavior. 2nd edition. Cambridge (UK): Cambridge University Press; 2000. p. 68–93.

[3] Lindell EM, Erb HN, Houpt KA. Intercat aggression: a retrospective study examining types of aggression, sexes of fighting pairs, and effectiveness of treatment. Appl Anim Behav Sci 1997;55:153–62.

[4] Horwitz DF, Neilson JC. Aggression/feline: redirected. In: Blackwell's five-minute veterinary consult clinical companion—canine & feline behavior. Ames (IA): Blackwell Publishing Professional; 2007. p. 148–54.

[5] Horwitz DF, Neilson JC. Aggression/feline: play related. In: Blackwell's five-minute veterinary consult clinical companion—canine & feline behavior. Ames (IA): Blackwell Publishing Professional; 2007. p. 141–7.

[6] Chon E. The effects of queen (Felis sylvestris)-rearing versus hand-rearing on feline aggression and other problematic behaviors. In: Mills D, Levine E, Landsberg G, et al,

editors. Current issues and research in veterinary behavioral medicine. Papers presented at the 5th Veterinary Behavior Meeting. West Lafayette (IN): Purdue University Press; 2005. p. 201–2.

[7] Schwartz B, Wasserman EA, Robbins SJ. Aversive control of behavior: punishment and avoidance. In: Psychology of learning and behavior. 5th edition. New York: W.W. Norton & Company, Inc.; 2002. p. 186–214.

[8] Crowell-Davis SL. Intercat aggression. Compend Contin Educ Vet 2007;29(9):541–6.

[9] Schwartz B, Wasserman EA, Robbins SJ. Pavlovian conditioning: basic phenomena. In: Schwartz B, Wasserman EA, Robbins SJ, editors. Psychology of learning and behavior. 5th edition. New York: W.W. Norton & Company, Inc.; 2002. p. 41–69.

[10] Overall KL. Feline elimination disorders. In: Clinical behavioral medicine for small animals. St. Louis (MO): Mosby-Year Book, Inc.; 1997. p. 174.

[11] Crowell-Davis SL. Human feet are not mice: how to treat human-directed feline aggression. Compend Contin Educ Vet 2007;29(8):483–6.

[12] Beaver BV. Feline grooming behavior. In: Feline behavior: a guide for veterinarians. Philadelphia: W.B. Saunders Company; 1992. p. 259.

[13] Crowell-Davis SL, Murray T. Azapirones. In: Veterinary psychopharmacology. Ames (IA): Blackwell Publishing Professional; 2006. p. 114.

[14] Overall KL. Feline aggression. In: Clinical behavioral medicine for small animals. St. Louis (MO): Mosby-Year Book, Inc.; 1997. p. 147.

[15] Horwitz DF, Neilson JC. Aggression/feline: status related. In: Blackwell's five-minute veterinary consult clinical companion—canine & feline behavior. Ames (IA): Blackwell Publishing Professional; 2007. p. 155–61.

[16] Center SA, Elston TH, Rowland PH, et al. Fulminant hepatic failure associated with oral administration of diazepam in 11 cats. J Am Vet Med Assoc 1996;209(3):618–25.

[17] Mealey KL, Peck KE, Bennett BS, et al. Systemic absorption of amitriptyline and buspirone after oral and transdermal administration to healthy cats. J Vet Intern Med 2004;18(1): 43–6.

[18] Ciribassi J, Luescher A, Pasloske KS, et al. Comparative bioavailability of fluoxetine after transdermal and oral administration to healthy cats. Am J Vet 2003;64(8):994–8.

ELSEVIER
SAUNDERS

Vet Clin Small Anim 38 (2008) 1145–1162

VETERINARY CLINICS
SMALL ANIMAL PRACTICE

Obtaining a Pet: Realistic Expectations

Amy Marder, VMD, CAAB[a],*, Margaret M. Duxbury, DVM[b]

[a]Center for Shelter Dogs, Animal Rescue League of Boston, 10 Chandler Street, Boston, MA 02117, USA
[b]Behavior Service, University of Minnesota, Veterinary Medical Center, College of Veterinary Medicine, 1365 Gortner Avenue, St. Paul, MN 55108, USA

Millions of dogs are surrendered to shelters each year, many because of behavior problems [1,2]. Undoubtedly, each of these dogs entered a family that had high hopes for its future. So what happened to dash those hopes? A study sponsored by the National Council on Pet Population Study and Policy (NCPPSP) found that, compared with dogs still in homes, relinquished dogs were more likely to be young (<2 years old); to be of mixed breeding; to have been obtained at little to no cost; or to have been obtained from a shelter, a friend, or a pet store [2]. The same study found that people relinquishing dogs lacked important basic knowledge about dogs, for example, that different breeds tend to exhibit different behaviors. These findings suggest that appropriate education could decrease the number of failed pet-human relationships. Preadoption counseling is a legitimate valuable service to offer prospective dog owners that can also have a profound impact on the well-being of dogs. Veterinarians can help prospective owners approach the selection process with realistic expectations. Armed with information about where to obtain a dog and with specific knowledge about how differences in the age, breed, and gender of the dog may affect their experience, owners are better positioned to begin a successful relationship with a new canine family member. Prospective dog owners may not know to look to veterinarians for preadoption counseling. This service can be promoted like any other new and valuable service, for example, in printed brochures, flyers, advertisements, and examination room posters and through community educational lectures. It is also important to talk to existing clients intentionally, who may be considering another dog without the clinician's knowledge.

MATCHING DOG TO HOUSEHOLD
Puppy Versus Adult
One of the first considerations for prospective pet owners is whether to get a puppy or an adult dog. In the NCPPSP study previously cited, overactivity, destructiveness, and house soiling were more common in relinquished dogs.

*Corresponding author. E-mail address: amarder@arlboston.org (A. Marder).

0195-5616/08/$ – see front matter
doi:10.1016/j.cvsm.2008.04.011

Relinquished dogs were also more likely to be young (<2 years old). Choosing an adult dog may allow owners to bypass many of the normal but undesirable puppy and juvenile behaviors that require patience and skill to manage. Conversely, choosing a puppy gives the owner more control over the experiences that have an impact on its future behavior, such as whether or not it is socialized to children. Many behavior problems that are rooted in the dog's genetics and early history do not become obvious until the dog reaches 1 to 3 years of age [3,4] People choosing an immature dog should be made aware that the dog they take into their home may change as it continues to develop. Knowledge of what the dog's parents were like, or whether the dog was well socialized, helps to predict its adult behavior. Someone considering a 4- to 5-year-old dog that is tolerant and social with children can be more assured that this behavior is likely to continue as long as the learning environment is stable.

Gender

Many people considering a pet dog would be well suited with a dog of either gender. Gender-based differences in behavior do exist, however. Male dogs are more likely to urine mark, mount dogs or people, and roam the neighborhood [5,6]. Certain types of aggression are seen more commonly in male dogs than in female dogs; these include fighting with other male dogs [5–7] and owner-directed aggression (formerly called dominance aggression) [7,8]. Other types of aggression, such as predatory- and fear-related aggression have no sexually dimorphic bias and occur in both genders [9]. Several studies found that reported dog bites to human beings are more likely to have been inflicted by male dogs, especially intact males [10,11]. One study found that small female dogs were most likely to have bitten a family member or other familiar person, however [12].

In a 1985 study based on predictions made by veterinarians and dog show judges, male dogs were thought to be more active and destructive, more likely to snap at children, and more likely to engage in territorial defense than female dogs [13]. They were also considered to be more playful. These same experts estimated that female dogs would be more affectionate and easier to train for house training and obedience. If we were to focus on just these reports, it would be a wonder that anyone would ever own a male dog. It is important to remember that these opinion-based (not observational data-based) reports simply suggest trends intended to be helpful to owners but that individual dogs may not follow trends. There is no assurance that an individual female pup is going to be easier to train or less aggressive than her male littermate. Gender-based differences may be more important for people considering a dog whose breed already ranks high in a particular trait that is also affected by gender. For example, someone considering a breed that rates high for the trait labeled "dominance over owner" could expect that an intact male dog would have the greatest chance of expressing that trait to its fullest.

Several of the behaviors seen more commonly in male dogs are modified by castration, including urine marking, roaming, mounting, and fighting with other dogs [5,6]. Castration may have some modifying effect on aggression to owners as well, though this is less well documented. Aggression between dogs in the same household occurs more frequently and more seriously among female-female pairs and least often between a male dog and a female dog in the same household [14]. Veterinarians should counsel families adding a second dog to choose a new dog of the opposite gender.

Breed or Breed Type

With hundreds of different registered and unregistered breeds and an exponential number of intentional or unintentional breed crosses available, the types of dogs or puppies available to choose from are enormous. Sadly, one of the most important features people use to choose a dog seems to be its appearance. This contributes to unrealistic expectations; for example, when a dog with a soft cuddly appearance has decidedly different behavior. Breeds vary in the tasks they were bred to accomplish. A dog bred for herding or for territorial defense brings those tendencies to a home environment. It is easy to see how mismatches might occur when people choose dogs without first learning about the breed history of that type of dog.

Without a veterinarian to guide them toward more scientifically based information, owners often rely on breed descriptions developed by breeders and breed registries. Many of those descriptions focus on the physical appearance of the dog. For example, in a quick Internet search of the American Kennel club (AKC) site describing different dog breeds, several hundreds to thousands of words on physical features may precede a small paragraph devoted to the temperament of the dogs. Many temperament descriptions use anthropomorphic terms to describe the breed in the best possible light or refer back to historic information about the breed's original use. Although original use information can be helpful, it may not provide a complete picture, because breed-typical behavior can change significantly within a few generations, depending on traits selected intentionally or unintentionally by breeders [15]. These factors make it difficult for owners to find useful information.

Certain aspects of personality (playfulness and curiosity, fearlessness, and sociability) differ among dogs of different breeds and also among dogs of the same breed [15]. These factors may influence a dog's success in the home, but knowing how requires interpretation, which may be subjective and beyond the capacity of the average client. Finding user-friendly objective information for clients about breed differences can be difficult. One source is work done by Hart and Hart [13]. The authors identified 13 key behavior characteristics that, in their view, were clearly and unambiguously labeled (eg, ease of house training, snapping at children.) They then surveyed small animal veterinarians and obedience judges regarding the relative scores of 56 different breeds and ranked them for easy comparison. This information is available in the scientific literature [13,16] and in book form for the lay public [17]. It is important to understand that these behavior profiles are based on the beliefs of veterinarians and judges and not on objective data collected by quantifying specific behaviors in specific dogs. Still, comparing information gained from breeders and breed registries with that found in the Harts' book may give prospective owners a more complete picture of a breed or breed combination that they are considering. For example, one terrier described on the AKC Web site as "alert, gay, courageous and self-reliant" was found in Harts' work to be in the highest percentile category for excitability, general activity level, snapping at children, excessive barking, watchdog barking, aggression toward other dogs, and destructiveness. Those with plenty of dog experience may read between the lines to see the same dog in both descriptions; however, without further education, many prospective owners may be misled.

When considering what breed is right, owners do well to consider their own life style and environment. The terrier from the previous example may be a poor choice for an inactive couple who live in a managed condominium with a small yard next to a busy sidewalk. Individuals of certain breeds, such as pointers, can have extremely high exercise requirements that require more than casual walks to satisfy. Households with children are inherently more challenging to manage. Families with children should be advised to choose a dog that is calmer and well socialized with children and individuals who are not members of the family because the dog has to interact safely with the children in addition to their friends and their friends' parents. Young couples should be advised to choose the same type of dog if they plan to have children and then ensure continued social exposure to children and unfamiliar people. The importance of proper socialization cannot be overemphasized (Box 1, Table 1).

SOURCE

Before owners decide where to look for a dog, they should ask themselves "why do I want to get a dog?" There is no right or wrong answer. Some people want a dog with a specific temperament and working ability or simply want to do everything right. For these owners, the more information they can gather before adoption, the better. Some owners are more relaxed about the outcome or want to give a disadvantaged dog a chance. These owners may expect less information and be comfortable with less control. Much depends on the risk tolerance of the prospective owner. The key is to have owners decide what they really want before they find themselves forced to choose whether to take or leave an attractive dog with a questionable background.

Purebred or Mixed Breed

Whether clients choose a mixed breed or purebred dog often depends on the answers to these questions. People who decide they want the most information and control often elect to purchase a purebred dog. These owners have a choice of sources, but are often unaware that the information, quality of care, and health or temperament assurances vary tremendously depending on whether they buy from a highly invested breeder, from a casual or "backyard" breeder, or from a breed production facility like a puppy mill or Internet sales operation.

Box 1: Optional list information for sidebars

Factors affecting adult behavior
- Genetic temperament
- Prenatal nutrition and maternal stress
- Early handling and socialization
- Interaction with littermates before adoption
- Quality and quantity of socialization experiences after adoption
- Learning experiences at any age
- Owner control of learning environment

Topics for preadoption counseling
- Avoid impulse purchases
- Registration papers, champions in pedigree, or designer breeding do not predict a "good" dog
- Goals for owning dog and degree of risk tolerance
- Considerations regarding source, breed, age, and gender
- Temperament tests are not predictive
- The "Rule of 3"
  - Look at multiple options
  - Make decision away from site to avoid situational social pressure

Red flags: beware if any of the following are noted
- Internet sales allowing you to pick and finalize a sale on-line
- Multiple breeds or breed mixes available from a single source
- Puppies marketed in retail stores
- Breeder offers to meet you in a parking lot for convenience
- Breeder who avoids having you visit the property
- Breeder who resents clients who ask questions
- Shy or timid parent; shy or timid puppy

Important points about socialization
- Puppies are most open to socialization between 3 and 12 weeks of age
- Social exposure should start at the breeders and continue throughout the dog's life
- Owners purchasing a 7- to 8-week-old puppy should start intentional socialization immediately
- Provide puppies with positive experiences with men, women, and children of all ages and ethnicities
- Provide puppies with positive experiences with dogs of different breeds and sizes
- Expose summer puppies to parkas, boots, and face masks
- Expose winter puppies to sunglasses, bicycles, rollerblades, and joggers
- Do not force shy puppies to interact; reduce the perceived threat and reward voluntary approach

Table 1
Shelter programs intended to reduce incidence of unrealistic expectations

Assessment	Benefits	Problems
Behavioral history	Identifies future house soiling, barking, destruction	Does not reliably identify aggressive behavior
Behavioral assessment	May identify future possessive behavior, defensive behavior, and mouthing	Unreliable predictor of many behaviors
Observations of daily behaviors	May identify some behaviors not evident on other assessments	Subject to staff opinions
Foster homes	Home environment may be more reliable predictor of behavior in adoptive home	Behavior affected by the presence of other dogs

Owners should be advised that registration papers or a pedigree full of champion ancestors does not predict that a puppy is going to be good if its temperament is not suitable. It should also be noted that there is nothing about the many so-called "designer" or planned mixed breeds that make them better than any other purebred or mixed-breed dog when little is known about the individual genetic backgrounds in the pedigree. Unless owners are willing to work to find highly invested breeders that can provide them with good information about the genetics and early environment of the puppies they produce, they may do just as well purchasing a mixed-breed puppy or an adult dog from a shelter.

Highly Invested Breeders

These breeders typically have specific breeding goals in mind for producing healthy dogs that are free of hereditary defects and also have specific conformation, working ability, and temperament. Meeting these goals requires that breeding stock undergo extensive testing for hereditary diseases, some of which cannot be completed until the dog is 2 years old. DNA testing has opened a new era in our ability to test for genetic diseases, further increasing the responsibility and expense for breeders working to produce healthy dogs. Highly invested breeders tend to be familiar with the particular traits of the individuals in the pedigree. In fact, they may own siblings, parents, aunts, and grandparents of a prospective litter, which represents a wonderful opportunity for prospective buyers to sneak a peek into the future; that is, if they like the relatives, chances are they are going to like the puppy. The best breeders would be aware of how early environmental factors influence the future behavior of the puppy and provide the bitch with good nutrition and a stable environment. Knowing that the important process of socialization begins under their watch, when the puppies are approximately 3 weeks old, they would also handle the puppies daily and expose them to novelty; to household sounds; and to unfamiliar people, including children, Purchasing a puppy from this type of breeder does not guarantee a successful outcome but may decrease the likelihood of unpleasant surprises. Puppies from these breeders are often expensive, because it costs money to screen for genetic defects and provide quality care and monitoring. Highly invested breeders can be choosy about where their dogs or puppies go. Prospective owners may need to meet certain requirements before purchase, usually having to do with the safety, well-being, and reproductive status of the dog. Veterinarians can encourage people to consider the cost of the dog in light of the years of enjoyment they hope to receive. Compared with other opportunities for companionship and entertainment, the costs for even a highly priced dog are minimal. Owners who spend more money on the dog seem to be less likely to relinquish that dog later [2].

"Casual" Breeders

Owners should learn the difference between highly invested breeders and more casual breeders who, for example, may simply own a "nice dog" and breed it to another. Each nice dog carries with it an extensive family history that may contain transmissible health or temperament defects not apparent in the individual. Inherited defects continue in breeds when they are not actively identified and selected against. People purchasing a puppy from a casual or backyard breeder may be able to evaluate the early environment and meet one or both parents but often gain no knowledge of the family tree behind each individual. These puppies may or may not be less expensive, but genetic testing is often lacking.

Breed Production and Sales Facilities

Some breeders simply produce a marketable commodity of purebred puppies without close regard for the effects of genetics and early environmental influences. These breeders can appear almost anywhere and may market several different breeds. People purchasing from pet stores support an industry whose goal too often is to sell puppies without concern about the outcome for the puppy or the owner as the puppy turns into a dog. Some pet stores purchase puppies from puppy mills that provide a less than optimum prenatal and early environment. Walking past an adorable puppy in a retail window may encourage impulsive buying from someone with no idea of what it takes to own a dog or that factors in its pedigree or early environment may be important. People considering a puppy they have found on-line should be aware that most reputable breeders do not sell puppies to people without having met and interviewed the prospective buyer. The Internet offers no protection against sellers who present themselves or their dogs inaccurately and, in these authors' opinion, is a poor place to buy a dog.

Shelters

Statistics on the human factors associated with pet relinquishment suggest that there are some nice dogs available in shelters—dogs whose first dog-human relationship failed simply because of the owner's lack of knowledge and commitment. Other dogs are relinquished to shelters because of true behavior problems that would persist in any home. The next section of this article focuses on what to consider when choosing a dog from a shelter or rescue group.

CHOOSING THE RIGHT PUPPY

Temperament Testing

Several temperament tests [18,19] have been designed to help match puppies to families. Unfortunately, research shows that formal temperament tests administered at 7 or 8 weeks of age do not successfully predict a puppy's future behavior [20–23]. Although clear differences in the way puppies score on these tests are apparent, the differences do not seem to be stable over time or predict how the puppy is going to react to specific situations that occur within households. Temperament tests have been used successfully to predict the success or failure of guide dogs undergoing training [24]. These tests were administered repeatedly over several weeks to months and through several stages of development, however, which is a situation that is not possible for most people purchasing a family dog. Dogs with a bold temperament seem to do better than dogs with a shy temperament in the number and variety of working dog trials, suggesting that whether a puppy is shy or bold may correlate with its overall trainability [25]. Given that fearfulness seems to be heritable [26], prospective owners would be wise to avoid choosing a puppy from shy parents or one that appears timid or fearful itself.

The "Rule of 3"

The juvenile physical characteristics of puppies are appealing to human beings, and this can lead to impulse purchases. Even people who have done some homework and decided on the age and breed of the dog they hope to get can impulsively choose the first puppy they see that fits the physical description. Veterinarians may have little chance to talk to owners before impulsive purchase opportunities unless they proactively counsel clients on the topic. Most owners do not scout out dog-purchasing options until they are buying a dog. If they only look at a single option, their ability to appreciate differences is negligible. Owners can gain helpful perspective if they promise themselves that they are not going to come home with a dog or puppy until they have explored at least three options. Visiting multiple breeders helps owners to appreciate differences among the breeding philosophies, the dogs themselves, and the environments in which the dogs are housed to determine the best "fit" before buying an adult dog or putting a deposit down on a puppy from a future litter. Owners can establish a list of behavior traits they consider important and use this list to create questions for interviewing different breeders. Veterinarians can provide information about genetic diseases common in certain breeds so that the owner can question the breeder appropriately. Owners should be counseled to beware of any breeder who discourages them from visiting their dogs and facilities, even if offered as a convenience, for example, to decrease the prospective purchaser's driving time.

Owners who are looking at purebred or mixed-breed litters on the ground or are choosing an adult dog can find the "look at 3" rule just as helpful. Most people benefit from having a chance to think about what they have seen and assess their true opinion without being influenced by the social pressures of the moment, such as the breeder expecting the owner to take a pup or the children vying for a different dog than the one the parents think is best. The recommendation to look at three different litters is easiest for owners to follow if the adults, the children, and the breeders or dog owners themselves know the plan ahead of time. Once a litter is selected, the "look at 3" rule can be applied to the number of times the owners visit the litter to look at individual puppies. The behavior of any individual pup may vary depending on the time of day of the visit and the recent feeding and activity level of each pup. An owner may choose a quiet puppy that only wants to snuggle in his or her lap without knowing that this same pup was a rocket on legs just a few minutes before his or her arrival. Owners should be cautious of litters in which either parent is timid or fails to approach them socially. Without prior education, owners may fail to recognize that the quiet puppy in the corner is actually shy and timid and not the ideal choice.

Shelter and Rescue Adoptions
Many people choose to adopt dogs from animal shelters and rescue groups (Fig. 1). Some prospective owners want to save a dog from possible euthanasia,

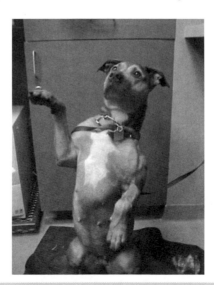

Fig. 1. American shelter dog.

whereas others are motivated to give the dog a better home than the one it previously inhabited. Still others adopt for economic reasons, because dogs from shelters and rescue groups tend to cost less than those from breeders and pet stores. Veterinarians are in a perfect position to counsel people who desire to "rescue" dogs so that they can find a suitable pet and are less likely to be disappointed by false expectations.

The advent of "Cybershelter" Web sites (Petfinder.com) has made shopping for a shelter or rescue dog relatively easy. Photographs and descriptions of dogs from all over the country are available for on-line viewing. People can search for the type of dog they desire (eg, age, breed) and fall in love on-line. If the dog is local, the potential adopters can meet the dog in a shelter or rescue home. People often choose and pay for dogs (especially puppies) who are located some distance away, however. In these cases, the new owners meet their dog only after it arrives at a local parking lot. Many groups transport dogs from areas of the country in which canine overpopulation is a severe problem (southern and midwest states) to areas in which there is a shortage of surplus dogs (northeastern states) Some rescue groups even import dogs from countries outside of the United States. Although many of the groups who transport dogs evaluate the dogs medically and behaviorally and vaccinate and neuter before transport, some do not. Veterinarians should be aware of the groups that are actively transporting dogs to their area and steer their clients toward the reputable groups and away from those that are not. Veterinarians can get some information on the reputability of transport groups through their state veterinarian or local humane society.

When advising a client where to go to find a well-matched shelter dog, and thus be less likely to be disappointed by false hopes, it is essential that veterinarians and potential adopters recognize that not all rescue groups are alike. They differ in their resources, funding, and organization. In general. shelters are free-standing buildings. Rescue groups may have their own shelters, use other shelters, or place their animals in foster homes. Some shelters are controlled by a municipality, whereas others are private. Some have a paid staff, and others are staffed completely by volunteers. Some groups are "no-kill" in that they try to save every animal received, sometimes housing multiple unadoptable animals. Others are "kill" in the sense that they euthanize some animals because they do not have enough room or resources to humanely care for the numbers of animals that enter their shelter. Some organizations are "limited admission" in that they do not admit "unadoptable" animals. Others are "open admission" in that they take in every animal in need. Some shelters admit only owner surrenders. Others admit strays, abandoned animals, and abused and neglected animals. In general, municipal shelters handle stray and abandoned animals, whereas many private shelters and rescue groups do not. Groups also have variable resources. The ideal organization has a shelter veterinarian on staff in addition to a behavior department; however, most do not. Many shelters neuter all animals before they are homed, and most of these practice early-age neutering. It is important for veterinarians to educate themselves regarding the capabilities and limitations of their local animal shelters and rescue groups. No matter the type of rescue group, however, clients should be directed to those that try to find out all they can about the behavior of the dogs they are placing and practice responsible matching. With the innovation of multiple behavioral assessment strategies, it is no longer acceptable for an adopter to be told that nothing is known about an individual dog. Through the acquisition of behavioral information on each dog, each potential new owner can be counseled about what to expect in their adopted pet. In this way, the hope is to limit unrealistic expectations, which often result in adoption failures (see Table 1).

Behavioral History

The collection of information about an individual dog begins with the person surrendering the animal, whenever possible. Of course, histories cannot be obtained on stray or abandoned animals. Many kinds of questionnaires are used by shelters to collect behavioral and medical histories on each animal. Although some are more objective than others, they are all subject to distortions in the subjective reports of owners. The surrender of an animal is an emotionally difficult decision for many owners. Because a person does not want to see his or her pet euthanatized, he or she may be biased (not truthful) in reporting past behavior. In addition, many owners relinquish after a brief period of time of owning their pets, resulting in an even more inaccurate behavioral history. Two studies have looked at the accuracy of behavioral histories [27,28]. Both have concluded that people are likely to hide aggressive tendencies in their dogs, whereas admitting to fearful behaviors, behaviors when left alone (eg, destruction, house soiling, barking), barking, and attention-seeking behaviors. One study found the intake information on these behaviors to be predictive of owner-reported behaviors 3 months after adoption. Therefore, although an intake history has its limitations, it is a worthwhile tool for collecting behavioral information.

Behavioral Evaluations

The next procedure used by shelters to assess a dog's behavioral tendencies is a formal behavioral evaluation (sometimes referred to as a "temperament test"), wherein a dog's responses to a variety of challenges are assessed (Fig. 2). Although there is little evidence [29] that these tests reliably predict behavior in a home environment after adoption, shelters choose to perform the tests so that they have more acceptable reasons for euthanasia. Often, these tests are given more value than a behavioral history. Because of the constraints of individual shelters (eg, space, number of animals, staff, staff training, staff bias), there is much variability in the types of tests used, their consistency, and their interpretation. Unfortunately, the rigorous reliability and validity testing required to confirm that a test is consistently answering the questions that are being asked is difficult or next to impossible to do in the shelter environment.

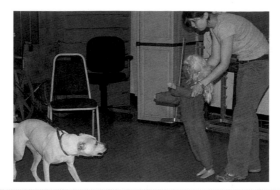

Fig. 2. Shelter agent behavioral testing a dog at the Animal Rescue League of Boston.

One of the most popular tests used in shelters is the "SAFER test" (The Safety Assessment for Evaluating Rehoming), developed by Emily Weiss, PhD [30]. The SAFER test consists of seven parts ("making friends," stare, sensitivity while grabbing skin, tag/chase, intertoe pinch, food aggression, and interdog aggression). The test was developed in a large shelter that needed to identify unadoptable dogs quickly, safely, and with as few staff members as possible. Therefore, the test is short and relatively simple to administer. The claimed "validation" of the test is subject to numerous problems, however. Many of the dogs chosen to be in the validation study were euthanized for health and space reasons. Of the dogs adopted, 23% were returned within days. Telephone follow-ups were done 2 weeks after adoption, hardly enough time for adjustment to a new home. Furthermore, the follow-up questions were vague. Finally, none of the dogs who were deemed unadoptable were followed up to assess the accuracy of their categorization.

Another popular behavioral evaluation test used by shelters is "Assess-a-Pet" developed by Sue Sternberg. This test takes 15 minutes to administer and consists of more parts than the SAFER test. Assess-a-Pet assesses a dog's sociability; dominance; play; prey drive; mental sensitivity; reaction to other dogs, strangers, and children; possessiveness over food; and response to being hugged. This method was deemed worthwhile to increase adoption safety and success based on the experience of the people who used it. Kelly Bollen attempted to validate this method on more than 2000 dogs who had received the tests. She found a correlation between aggressive responses on the evaluation and reported aggressive behavior in the dog's previous home. She also found that if a dog displayed "borderline" behavior during the evaluation, the dog was more likely to show "problematic behavior" after adoption. The fact that both the evaluations and follow-ups were done by a single person makes these results subject to experimenter bias and is a severe flaw in experimental design [31].

Marder and Engel [32] at the American Society for the Prevention of Cruelty to Animals (ASPCA) conducted a study to determine whether any of 140 tests were predictive of behavior after adoption of 70 dogs aged 4 months and older. All the dogs evaluated were placed into homes. The tests chosen were things that owners were likely to do in the home (eg, petting, leaving alone, wiping feet, pushing into a sit, holding muzzle, touching food or dog while eating, pulling on collar, meeting a stranger, being reprimanded, being awakened while in a bed). The tests were performed by trained staff members, and evaluators recorded direct observations of the dog's behavior. Observations were then classified into the functional categories of fear, friendliness, arousal, or aggression. A 60-item questionnaire was administered to owners by telephone by one trained interviewer at 1 week, 1 month, 2 months, 3 months, and 6 months after adoption. Each behavioral category (eg, possessive aggression, defensive aggression, aggression to other dogs) from the evaluation was compared with owner reports of similar behaviors after adoption. When the tests were compared using likelihood coefficients, the following tests were moderately predictive when positive: showing teeth; growling; snapping; or biting over food, rawhide, or sleeping area predicted similar possessive aggression in the home. Showing teeth, growling, snapping, or biting a threatening person predicted aggression to strangers after adoption, and mouthing during the evaluation predicted mouthing in the home. On the negative side, only the absence of friendliness was moderately predictive of not being friendly. The other tests were mildly predictive or not predictive at all. Like the other follow-up studies, this one also has serious flaws. Interrater reliability among the evaluators was not tested, and owner reporting was used. Nevertheless, the results of this study suggest that many tests done routinely in shelters to assess adoptability and suitability for euthanasia are, at best, only weak predictors of behavior after adoption.

Because of the lack of reliable tests at this time, the behavioral evaluation should be considered as only one of the tools used to predict future behavior in choosing appropriate homes for adopted animals. The information gleaned from these evaluations should also be judiciously used in counseling potential adopters about realistic expectations. Fortunately, numerous studies are now in progress to develop better methods of predicting dogs' behavior.

Behavioral Observations in Shelter or Foster Home

More accurate predictions regarding future behavior may result from the observation of a dog's behavior in a temporary home. Many rescue groups use foster homes to house dogs before adoption. Although each home environment differs in terms of its human and animal residents, the confinement and stress of the shelter is eliminated, allowing the dog to feel safe and express less self-protective behaviors. Some shelters use offices and "real-life" rooms to imitate homes to get a better view of the dog's behavior.

While housed in the shelter or a temporary home, records of the dog's daily behavior in reaction to different people and environments may reveal important information that may not be apparent on the intake or thorough behavioral evaluation. Fears of noises, chasing behavior, and predatory behavior are good examples of behaviors that are often missed in other types of evaluations. Furthermore, a dog's behavior may change over time in the shelter or temporary home. Therefore, knowledge of a dog's daily behavior is essential to understand a dog's behavioral tendencies and to provide potential adopters with realistic expectations.

Making Matches

After the behavioral information on each dog is obtained and the dog is deemed suitable for adoption (suitability differs among organizations), the best-matched home is then sought. Most organizations have potential adopters complete applications and participate in an interview to determine the characteristics of the family. The matching process is quite variable among shelters. "Meet Your Match, Canine-ality," a program designed by Emily Weiss, PhD, is a formal matching program now used by many shelters. It consists of a series of behavioral tests for each dog and a questionnaire for potential owners. Dogs and owners are classified and given a color-coded card. Owners are urged to only look at the dogs that match their colors.

The Animal of Rescue League of Boston uses the "Sneak-a-Peek" dog description and owner application (Fig. 3) designed by Amy Marder, VMD. Based on the results of a behavioral assessment, an evaluator completes the dog's Sneak-a Peek, which describes the requirements of a potential adoptive home for each dog. Requirements include experience of owners, exercise, ages of family members, other animals in the household, grooming needs, ease of training, crating recommendations, and house training. The list of requirements is placed on each dog's cage to be viewed by potential adopters. Every adopter, in turn, fills out an application with questions that directly pertain to each of the requirements. Using this device, adoption counselors direct adopters to appropriate animals. Adopters are dissuaded from choosing dogs based on appearance alone and are counseled to attend closely to the dog's behavioral needs.

Individual shelters claim that after using matching programs they have experienced a reduction in return-to-shelter rates. No accumulation of data across shelters has been done, however.

The ASPCA follow-up after the behavioral evaluation indicated that the most common problems after adoption were house soiling, destruction, and barking. House soiling and barking as problem behaviors significantly reduced over time. By 3 months after adoption, they were infrequent. Dogs most likely go through an adjustment period to their new homes; during this time, their behavior changes. Destruction did not change significantly over the 3-month period. Aggression to strangers and fear of people increased significantly between 2 and 3 months after adoption. Aggression to family members did not change over time.

Veterinarians can help in the process by recommending shelters that do thorough intakes, behavior evaluations, observation of behavior, and follow-up, all of which help to decrease the incidence of false expectations.

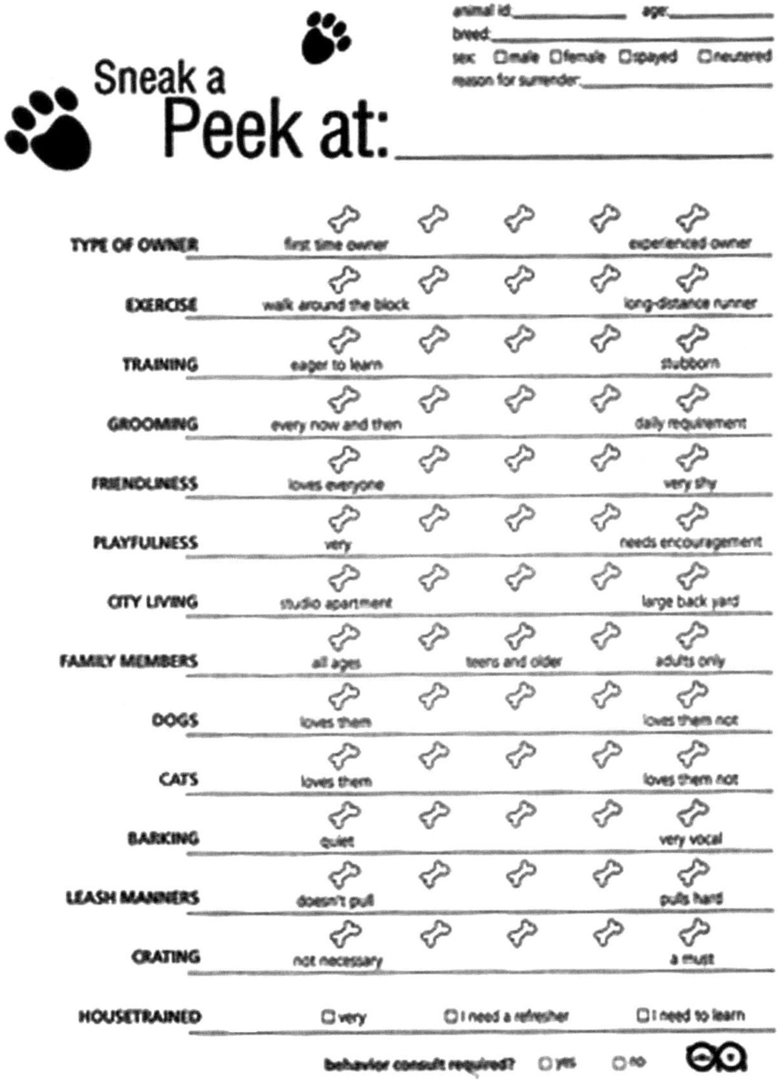

Sneak a
Peek at: _____

animal id _____ age: _____
breed: _____
sex: ☐ male ☐ female ☐ spayed ☐ neutered
reason for surrender: _____

| TYPE OF OWNER | first time owner | | | | experienced owner |
| GROOMING | every now and then | | | | daily requirement |

TYPE OF OWNER — first time owner / experienced owner

EXERCISE — walk around the block / long-distance runner

TRAINING — eager to learn / stubborn

GROOMING — every now and then / daily requirement

FRIENDLINESS — loves everyone / very shy

PLAYFULNESS — very / needs encouragement

CITY LIVING — studio apartment / large back yard

FAMILY MEMBERS — all ages / teens and older / adults only

DOGS — loves them / loves them not

CATS — loves them / loves them not

BARKING — quiet / very vocal

LEASH MANNERS — doesn't pull / pulls hard

CRATING — not necessary / a must

HOUSETRAINED — ☐ very   ☐ I need a refresher   ☐ I need to learn

behavior consult required?   ☐ yes   ☐ no

Fig. 3. Animal Rescue League of Boston "Sneak-a-Peek." (*Courtesy of* Animal Rescue League of Boston, Boston, MA; with Permission.)

Importantly, the veterinarian should be cognizant of the difficulty in the process and, after seeing an adopted dog, should not criticize the shelter or rescue group. The diagnosis of behavior problems in dogs from shelters and rescue groups is no different than that of behavior problems in dogs from breeders. Instead, put in place resources to help counsel the new owner about behavior issues and offer good resources for treatment of behavior problems (see Table 1).

Postadoption Follow-Up and Outcome Measures

The success of each program designed to reduce the incidence of unrealistic expectations and increase the success of adoptions can be determined only by measuring outcome results. Many shelters are computerized and routinely record the number of animals returned to their shelters. Success is claimed by a reduction in the percentage of animals returned. These numbers are only a partial indicator of adoption success, however, because many people who do not keep their animals give them to friends or relatives, or, in worst cases, allow them to stray. Shelters who do regular follow-ups on their adoptions can more accurately claim success based on the numbers of animals that stay in their adoptive homes. Follow-ups also allow shelters to advise people on behavioral problems that occur after adoption. Many shelters also have behavior help lines, but there are no good data available as to their usefulness in retention of adopted animals. Unfortunately, many surveys have indicated that the most likely thing that owners do about behavior problems is nothing or calling a dog trainer, whereas cat owners do nothing or call a behavior consultant. Offering behavior services within the veterinary practice might help these individuals to find the help they need.

SUMMARY

Choosing a future family pet is a personal and important decision. The dog that one person considers a perfect companion may be "all wrong" for another potential owner. Veterinarians can provide a real service to clients by offering preadoption counseling to help them sort through the many factors involved in the process of successful pet selection and by preparing them to take on the important task of socializing the puppy and managing its learning environment once it arrives in the home.

Veterinarians can have a large role in making adoptions successful. First, they can advise their clients to go to shelters or rescue groups that have programs designed to reduce the incidence of unrealistic expectations and have follow-up interviews to test the success of their programs. Some shelters also offer help lines for new adopters to aid in resolutions of problems after adoption. Then, because of their unique position of seeing newly adopted animals soon after adoption, veterinarians can take the time to provide behavioral education, explain misconceptions, identify and discuss behavioral problems, and recommend obedience training. The support given to a new owner of a shelter dog during this important time of relationship building may ensure that the animal stays in the new home. Whether by aiding owners in the selection of a dog, preparing new owners to take on the task of socializing a puppy and managing its learning environment once in the home, or educating owners on the needs and behaviors of adult dogs, veterinarians can play a crucial role in making adoptions successful.

References

[1] New JC, Salman MD, Scarlett JM, et al. Moving: characteristics of dogs and cats and those relinquishing them to 12 U.S. animal shelters. J Appl Anim Welf Sci 1999;(2):83–96.

[2] New JC, Salman MD, King M, et al. Characteristics of shelter-relinquished animals and their owners compared with animals and their owners in U.S. pet-owning households. J Appl Anim Welf Sci 2000;(3):179–201.

[3] Beaver BV. Canine behavior. Philadelphia: WB Saunders; 1999. p. 157.

[4] Bowen J, Heath S. Behaviour problems in small animals: practical advice for the veterinary team. Philadelphia: Elsevier; 2005. p. 121.

[5] Hart BL. Effects of neutering and spaying on the behavior of dogs and cats: questions and answers about practical concerns. J Am Vet Med Assoc 1981;198:1204–5.

[6] Hopkins SG, Schubert TA, Hart BL. Castration of adult male dogs: effects on roaming, aggression, urine marking and mounting. J Am Vet Med Assoc 1976;168:1108–10.

[7] Borchelt PL, Voith VL. Dominance aggression in dogs. In: Voith PL, Borchelt PL, editors. Readings in companion animal behavior. New Jersey: Veterinary Learning Systems; 1996. p. 235.

[8] Reisner IR. Differential diagnosis and management of human-directed aggression in dogs. Vet Clin North Am Small Anim Pract 2003;33(2):304.

[9] Voith VL, Borchelt PL. Aggression in dogs and cats. In: Voith PL, Borchelt PL, editors. Readings in companion animal behavior. New Jersey: Veterinary Learning Systems; 1996. p. 222.

[10] Borchelt PL. Aggressive behavior of dogs kept as companion animals: classification and influence of sex, reproductive status and breed. Appl Anim Ethol 1983;10:45–61.

[11] Wright JC, Nesselrote MS. Classification of behavior problems in dogs: distribution of age, breed, sex and reproductive status. Appl Anim Behav Sci 1987;19:169–78.

[12] Guy NC, Luescher UA, Dohoo SE, et al. Risk factors for dog bites to owners in a general veterinary caseload. Appl Anim Behav Sci 2001;74:29–42.

[13] Hart BL, Hart LA. Selecting pet dogs on the basis of cluster analysis of breed behavior profiles and gender. J Am Vet Med Assoc 1985;186:1181–5.

[14] Sherman CK, Reisner IR, Taliaferro LA, et al. Characteristics, treatment and outcome of 99 cases of aggression between dogs. Appl Anim Behav Sci 1996;(47):91–108.

[15] Svartberg K. Breed-typical behaviour in dogs—historical remnants or recent constructs? Appl Anim Behav Sci 2006;(96):293–313.

[16] Hart BL, Miller MF. Behavioral profiles of dog breeds: a quantitative approach. J Am Vet Med Assoc 1985;186(11):1175–80.

[17] Hart BL, Hart LA. The perfect puppy: how to choose your dog by its behavior. New York: WH Freeman; 1988.

[18] Volhard W, Volhard J. Puppy Aptitude Test.

[19] Campbell WE. A behavior test for puppy selection. Mod Vet Pract 1972;53:29–33.

[20] Reid PJ, Penny N, et al. Predicting canine behaviour through early assessment. In: Overall KL, Mills DS, Heath SE, editors. Proceedings of the Third International Congress on Veterinary Behavioural Medicine. UK: Universities Federation for Animal Welfare; 2001. p. 92–5.

[21] Wilsson E, Sundgren PE. Behavior test for eight week old puppies—heritabilities of tested behaviour traits and its correspondence to later behaviour. Appl Anim Behav Sci 1998;(58):151–62.

[22] Beaudet R, Chalifoux A, Dallaire A. Predictive value of activity level and behavioural evaluation on future dominance in puppies. Appl Anim Behav Sci 1994;(40):273–84.

[23] Jones AC, Gosling SD. Temperament and personality in dogs (Canis familiaris): a review and evaluation of past research. Appl Anim Behav Sci 2005;(95):1–53.

[24] Goddard ME, Beilharz RG. Early prediction of adult behavior in potential guide dogs. Appl Anim Behav Sci 1986;(15):247–60.

[25] Svartberg K. Shyness-boldness predicts performance in working dogs. Appl Anim Behav Sci 2002;(79):157–74.

[26] Overall KA. Clinical behavioral medicine for small animals. St. Louis (MO): Mosby; 1997. p. 43–44.

[27] Segurson SA, Serpell JA, et al. Evaluation of a behavioral assessment questionnaire for use in the characterization of behavioral problems of dogs relinquished to animal shelters. J Am Vet Med Assoc 2005;227(11):1755–61.

[28] Marder AR, Ehrman R. A comparison of canine behavior in pre-adoptive and post-adoptive homes [poster]. In: Proceedings of the 5th International conference on Veterinary Behavioral Medicine; Minneapolis (MN).

[29] Reid P, Goldman J, et al. Animal shelter behavior programs. In: Miller L, Zawistowski S, editors. Shelter medicine for veterinarians and staff. Ames (IA): Blackwell; 2004. p. 317–31.

[30] Weiss E. Safer: the safety assessment for evaluating and rehoming. Engelwood (CO): American Humane; 2001.

[31] Dowling J. Putting your behavior evaluation program to the test. Animal Sheltering Sept–Oct 2003.

[32] Marder AR, Engel JM. Predictability of a shelter dog assessment test [abstract]. In: Proceedings of the 1st Annual Meeting of the American College of Veterinary Behaviorists.

INDEX

0195-5616/08/$ – see front matter
doi:10.1016/S0195-5616(08)00145-9